Applied

Microbiology

Applied
Microbiology

EDITED BY

Pam Caddow

RGN, RSCN, RM, DipN (Lond)
In-Patient Services Manager,
Barnet General Hospital

SCUTARI PRESS

© Scutari Press 1989

A division of Scutari Projects, the publishing
company of the Royal College of Nursing

First published 1989

British Library Cataloguing in Publication Data
Applied microbiology
   1. Medicine. Microbiology
   I. Caddow, Pam
   616′.01

   ISBN 1-871364-08-6

Typeset by MC Typeset Limited, Gillingham, Kent
Printed and bound in Great Britain by
The Alden Press Oxford London and Northampton

Contributors

Betty Bowell, RFN, RGN, ONC, SCM, DipN, RCNT, Clinical Nurse Advisor, Bath Health Authority

Pam Caddow, RGN, RSCN, RM, DipN(Lond), In-Patient Services Manager, Barnet General Hospital

Glenys Griffiths, RGN, SCM, FAETC, Senior Nurse – Infection Control, Mayday Hospital, Croydon, Chairman of the London Group of the ICNA

Kate Phillips, BA, SRN, RMN, SCM, Nurse Advisor, Department of Service Evaluation and Development, Bloomsbury Health Authority, London

Stephen Potter, MSc, MCPP, MRPharmS, Principal Pharmacist, Queen Elizabeth Hospital, Birmingham

Diane Thomlinson, BSc, SRN, ONC, Senior Nurse, Infection Control, Worcester Royal Infirmary, Worcester

'A rotten apple in the barrel contaminating the rest has some similarities with a hospital. Failure to recognise a bad apple or to appreciate its importance when packing the barrel can initiate the problems. After this the size of the barrel and how full it is will determine the number of apples that can become bad. Checking the apples and removing bad ones may stop the process spreading and spraying or wrapping the apples or dividing the barrel into sections may reduce the number of casualties. The design of the barrel and how well it is maintained can also have some effect. However, failures in managing storage are usually more important. Complaining about the barrel without taking any other action will not save the apples.' (From Collins B, 1981, *Nursing*, **29**, 9)

Contents

Preface

'Applied Microbiology' is a handbook for health-care workers which aims to give microbiological information in a form which can be used in a problem-solving approach to every-day situations.

The text has mostly been prepared by practising infection control nurses who are in the unique position of working with all grades and all disciplines of health authority personnel. While this book addresses the need for a multidisciplinary commitment to infection control, we anticipate that our principal readers will be nurses. The text has been prepared to enable nurses to participate in rational and informed individualised care.

We, the authors, have aimed to:

- Put microbiology into an historical perspective (chapter 1)
- Present a package of essential microbiology based on the clear identification of microbial behaviour patterns (chapter 2)
- Explain the physiology of the infection process and the body's normal and abnormal responses (chapter 3)
- Present the facts and realities of hospital- and community acquired infection (chapter 4)
- Define the parameters of the prevention and control of infection, and examine the respective contributory roles of people and the environment (chapter 5)
- Outline the role of the laboratory and discuss the relevance of correct specimens and the interpretation of laboratory reports (chapter 6)
- Explain the properties and potential problems of antimicrobial chemotherapeutic agents (chapter 7)
- Apply microbiology to the nursing process with a view to replacing the routine dangling of an isolation card on the door with the application of common sense (chapter 8)
- Give an insight into the scale and realities of pandemic epidemiology and infection (chapter 9)
- Consider the current trends in infection and communicable disease (chapter 10)

While it is outside the brief of a microbiology book, an appendix on parasitic skin infestation has been included as questions relating to this subject are frequently fielded by infection control personnel.

We have tried to make the text practical, and have attempted to make the book relevant, interesting and readable. Wherever possible, we have reinforced the information with case studies as nurses remember people for whom they have cared. We also hope that, while the core information (e.g. the behaviour of a specific organism) remains constant, the reader will see from the case studies how variables and risk factors such as age, morbidity and invasive procedures can positively or adversely affect the outcome for the patient; infection control nursing probably has more scope for individualised care than has any other field of nursing.

Information given in the text has been substantiated by references to research. For enquiring minds, we have concluded each chapter with a suggested further reading list. This book is a foundation text, and we hope that those who are interested will be encouraged to explore beyond its scope.

We would like to extend our thanks to the following for their help in preparation of the text: Sharon Burns, Mike Gill, Peter Hoffman, Carol Joseph and all at Scutari Press. On a personal note, I would like to thank Mark and Emma for their patience during my work on this manuscript.

Pam Caddow

1

Microbiology – An Historical

Backdrop

The control of infection is a responsibility shared by all disciplines working in the NHS although, through their regular 'hands on' contact with patients, nurses stand in the front line. In the UK, nurses are encouraged to use a reasoned, problem-solving approach to nursing, known as the nursing process, which is divided into four basic elements:

- Assessment
- Planning
- Implementation
- Evaluation

The nursing process is a very practical way of individualising care. The prevention and control of infection is an integral part of individualised patient care which needs to be addressed when applying the nursing process. For example, the initial assessment of an individual patient should include his risk of infection.

Infection control is too often regarded as an optional extra activity of care. Hospital-acquired infection (HAI) is frequently discussed as of little importance or as an inevitable accompaniment of hospital life (Worsley, 1983). The fact that HAI is not always included in the medical training curriculum shows how little importance is often attached to it, but it must be remembered that infection control is everybody's responsibility and everyone needs to participate.

Participants need to know what is required of them so must have some fundamental knowledge. Rationale is based on fundamental knowledge, and effective work practice is based on rationale. Western man has been slow to develop rationale in the field of microbiology, and a dip into the history books may help us to appreciate why this is.

Before medical science developed, the supernatural forces of good and evil were held accountable for illness. Disease was associated with the Devil or thought to be a punishment from the gods, while good health was believed to demonstrate approval of the good spirits or of God. However, some sort of infection control was being practised as long ago as 2000 BC.

2000 BC

When Europeans were still living in mud huts, King Hammurabi of Babylonia introduced public health measures into Babylon (Coleman, 1985). Clothes worn by people suffering from infectious diseases had to be burnt and the dead had to be carried far away from populated areas. Cattle had to be kept at a specified distance from houses. Dropping bones or refuse on the ground was punishable. Regulations protected water supplies from contamination and lavatories, drains and clean water supplies were in use. A highly organised medical profession was governed by strict rules and regulations. As Hastings (1974) tells us, physicians' remuneration was variable.

● 'If a physician has treated a nobleman for a severe wound with a bronze lancet and has cured him, or opened a nobleman's eye abscess and has cured it, he shall take 10 shekels of silver. If he be a freeman he shall receive five shekels. If the patient is a slave his master shall pay two shekles of silver . . . if the physician shall kill the patient or destroy the sight of the eye his hands shall be cut off . . .'

In India circa 2000 BC surgery was remarkably well developed (Coleman, 1985). The ancient Hindu surgeons used scalpels, scissors, hooks, probes, forceps, catheters and syringes. Operating theatres were kept scrupulously clean and the risk of cross-infection by contact was reduced by the surgeons scrubbing their hands and keeping their nails short. Clean, white clothing was worn in the operating theatre. The use of heat as an infection control measure was recognised and, as a result, sheets were steam-cleaned and instruments boiled. Operating rooms were well-lit and ventilated.

There is evidence to suggest that at this time the Indians and Chinese knew how to protect themselves against smallpox by inoculation. Ritual practices developed, such as the breaking of the skin between the thumb and forefinger to implant infected material from a smallpox pustule (McGrew, 1985). It was also appreciated that the use of mosquito netting could prevent malaria, an association that was not acknowledged by Western doctors until 1898.

ANCIENT GREECE

The founder of medical science, the Greek physician Hippocrates, was born in 460 BC. He dissociated medicine from religion and philosophy and established it as a separate scientific discipline. When looking for the cause of disease he would examine patients' environments – their home, work, etc. Through accurate observation of his patients, Hippocrates concluded that recovery of good health necessitated the supporting of the body's self-healing mechanisms. At this time, surgery was performed with unsterile instruments, but cleanliness was observed and surgeons pre-operatively pared their nails and cleansed their hands.

When Hippocrates died at the age of 99 years, medical progress halted. The Greek empire began to weaken and its decline was hastened when infection, in the form of plague, struck Athens. Power then passed to the Roman empire.

THE INFLUENCE OF ROME

The Romans contributed little to medicine but, being a practical people, they contributed enormously to the advancement of public health (Hastings, 1974), for instance by realising that disease was caused by filth and overcrowding. Zealous engineers in Rome designed an underground system of sewers, water-flush closets and public lavatories. By the second century AD, fresh water was channelled into Rome via 14 aqueducts which supplied the city with 300 million gallons of drinking water daily (figure 1.1). The homes of the wealthy had piped water and settling tanks to keep the water clean. Legislation was introduced to control street cleanliness, food hygiene and cremation of bodies, and hospitals were set up for the sick.

Travelling messengers and diplomats reporting to Rome carried with them not only news but also previously unknown diseases from abroad. These diseases included smallpox and measles, against which there was no immunity in the Roman

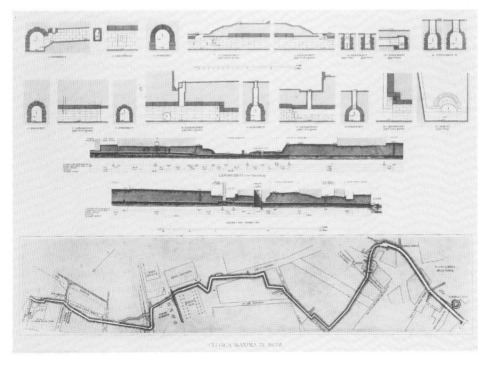

Fig 1.1   The cloaca maxima in Rome
(Reproduced by kind permission of the Wellcome Institute Library, London)

population. When the Roman drainage system fell into disuse following the Gothic invasions, the fields became swamps which in turn became breeding grounds for mosquitoes. Malaria, smallpox and measles killed thousands, and Roman standards of health gradually deteriorated.

THE MIDDLE AGES

The focus of medical development moved during the Middle Ages to the Arab world. The Arabs revived classical learning and continued the Roman system of hospitals, and also recognised epidemic fevers. The physician Rhezes used animal gut for suturing wounds. A textbook of surgery was produced by Albucasis of Cordova (936–1013 AD) in which he succinctly observed:

● 'Surgical operations are of two kinds, those which benefit the patient and those which kill him'.

The two most prevalent diseases in mediaeval times were leprosy and bubonic plague. Leprosy is well described in the Bible:

● '. . . and the leper in whom the plague is, his clothes shall be rent, and his head bare, and he shall put a covering upon his upper lip, and shall cry Unclean, Unclean. All the days wherein the plague shall be in him he shall be defiled; he is unclean; he shall dwell alone; without the camp shall his habitation be'. (Leviticus 13:45–46)

Lepers were believed to have transgressed against God, and were isolated from society and proclaimed dead as citizens. Special 'leper houses' were built outside the towns to isolate the victims from the community; in 1200 AD, about 19 000 leprosaria existed in the Christian countries. On special days, lepers were permitted to beg from house to house, being preceded by a warning bell. They were allowed to witness the holy ceremony of the Sacrament from outside, watching through the low side-windows often built into mediaeval parish churches.

Leprosy ceased to be a major disease at the close of the fourteenth century, only to be superseded by bubonic plague (the 'Black Death'). The causative bacillus, *Yersinia pestis*, was transmitted by rat fleas, producing swollen lymph glands in the armpits and groin (**buboes**). The Black Death was the disease's pneumonic form, a lethal infection which caused gangrene of the lungs. It was transmitted as easily then as a common cold is today. Bubonic plague is estimated to have killed about one third of the total population of Europe; in England alone 1.4 million people died of the disease (Zeigler, 1969).

The source of the outbreak was central Asia, where a natural disaster had caused the rats to desert their waterside homes and move to more populated areas. When these rats died, their fleas transferred to human Chinese hosts. By 1346 AD, plague had infected a Tartar army laying seige to the Genoese trading port of Kaffa on the Russian shore of the Black Sea. There followed the first recorded episode of biological warfare when the Tartars catapulted infected corpses over the city wall to infect their enemies. The Genoese left the city, taking the plague to northern Europe, while the Tartars carried it on to Russia, India and China (Coleman, 1985).

Many cures were proposed for bubonic plague, such as avoiding hard-boiled eggs, bathing the hands in vinegar or rose-water and keeping goats in the sufferer's bedroom. Vigorous activities like lovemaking, arguments and hot baths were to be avoided, which was unfortunate as the plague bacillus cannot survive extremes of temperature.

When treating victims of bubonic plague, doctors wore cloth helmets and respirators stuffed with herbs in an attempt to protect themselves (figure 1.2). Crosses were chalked on the doors of houses where victims lay dying, and bonfires were built in the streets. Efforts to prevent travellers bringing the plague into towns established the quarantine system when Eastern traders and immigrants seeking entry to Venice were isolated on a nearby island for forty days (quaranta giorni). This period of time – 40 days and 40 nights – was chosen because it was the duration of Christ's isolation in the wilderness.

In 1665, an epidemic of plague, unprecedented in size, broke out in London (figure 1.3). The plague bacillus was not isolated until 1894, and the theory that the bacillus was carried by man, fleas or rats was not finally substantiated until 1914. In 1665, dogs were suspected of spreading the outbreak, so four thousand of them were destroyed. This left the bacillus-carrying rats free to roam unmolested.

It was rumoured that tobacco and syphilis afforded protection against the plague, so tobacconists and prostitution flourished. Huge bonfires lit to dispel the 'plague venom' attracted dense crowds, which in turn increased the incidence of contact spread of the deadly infection. It is estimated that over one fifth of London's population died before the epidemic abated after the Great Fire of London in 1666. Also at this time, the resident black rats were driven out by incoming brown Norwegian rats which avoid humans.

A notable advance in microbiology was made in 1675 by Antony van Leeuwenhoek (1632–1723), a Dutch merchant and naturalist, who was the first man to see bacteria under one of the self-made microscopes which were his hobby (Hastings, 1974). After examining scales scraped from his feet, he wrote that he saw 'little animals more numerous than all people in the Netherlands and moving about in a most delightful manner'. Many people at the time believed that these 'animalcules' might be the cause of contagious disease, but this theory was not established as scientific fact until two hundred years later.

THE EIGHTEENTH CENTURY

A further advance was made in the eighteenth century when John Pringle (1707–1782), physician to the British Army, suspected that dirt might cause disease (Hastings, 1974). He introduced hygiene into army hospitals and first coined the word 'antiseptic'. Hospital personnel, however, continued to run the risk of acquiring an infection, and quite a risk that was, as the following passage describes.

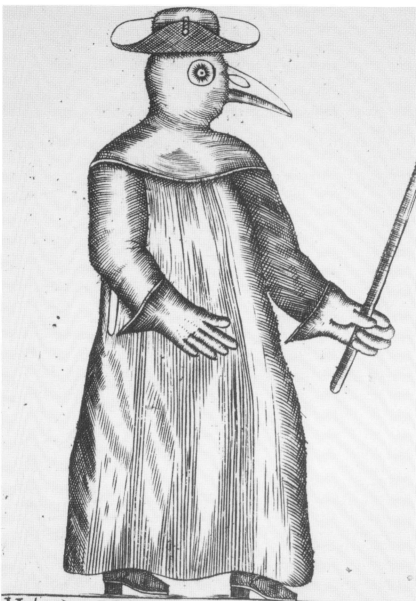

Habit des Medecins, et autres personnes qui visitent les Pestiferés, Il est de marroquin de leuant, le masque a les yeux de cristal, et un long néz rempli de parfums

Fig 1.2 Doctors' costumes during the Plague
(Reproduced by kind permission of the Wellcome Institute Library, London)

. The Diseases and Casualties this Week.

	Imposthume — 8
	Infants — 22
	Kingsevil — 4
	Lethargy — 1
	Livergrown — 1
	Meagrome — 1
	Palsie — 1
Abortive — 4	Plague — 4237
Aged — 45	Purples — 2
Bleeding — 1	Quinsie — 5 *
Broken legge — 1	Rickets — 23
Broke her scull by a fall in the street at St. Mary Woolchurch — 1	Rising of the Lights — 18
	Rupture — 1
Childbed — 28	Scurvy — 3
Chrisomes — 9	Shingles — 1
Consumption — 126	Spotted Feaver — 166
Convultion — 89	Stilborn — 4
Cough — 1	Stone — 2
Dropsie — 53	Stopping of the stomach — 17
Feaver — 348	Strangury — 3
Flox and Small-pox — 11	Suddenly — 2
Flux — 1	Surfeit — 74
Frighted — 2	Teeth — 111
Gowt — 1	Thrush — 6
Grief — 3	Tissick — 9
Griping in the Guts — 79	Ulcer — 1
Head-mould-shot — 1	Vomiting — 10
Jaundies — 7	Wind — 4
	Wormes — 20

Christned { Males — 90, Females — 81, In all — 171 } Buried { Males — 2777, Females — 2791, In all — 5568 } Plague — 4237

Increased in the Burials this Week — 249

Parishes clear of the Plague — 27 Parishes Infected — 103

The Assize of Bread set forth by Order of the Lord Maior and Court of Aldermen, A penny Wheaten Loaf to contain Nine Ounces and a half, and three half-penny White Loaves the like weight.

Fig 1.3 A bill of mortality for the week 15–22 August 1655, at the time of the Plague (Reproduced by kind permission of the Wellcome Insitute Library, London)

● 'January 1st 1770. A nurse in the fever ward of the infirmary, having several patients under her care, caught the infection. She was seized with violent rigors, chilliness and wandering pains, succeeded by great heat, thirst and headache. Sixteen hours after the first attack, her heat in the axilla [armpit] was 103° of fah [fahrenheit], her pulse 112 in the minute and strong, her thirst great, her tongue furred and her skin dry. Five gallons of salt water, of the temperature of 44° were poured over her naked body, at five o'clock in the afternoon, and after being hastily dried with towels, she was replaced in bed, when the agitation and sobbing had subsided heat and headache were gone, and the thirst nearly gone. Six hours afterwards she was found perfectly free of fever, but a good deal of debility remained.' (Williams, 1975)

The prisons of the day also provided ideal conditions for the spread of typhus, known as 'gaol fever' because it was widespread among the prison population. The vector of infection is the human body louse, but the court judges of the day believed that the source of the infection was the miasma or vapour which the prisoners emitted. In an attempt to avoid the risk of infection, some judges barricaded themselves behind huge bunches of flowers; this is the origin of today's custom of judges carrying a nosegay into court. Certainly the law courts were places of high risk in the spread of typhus fever (Hastings, 1974): in 1750, a hearing at London's Old Bailey was followed by the demise of the city's Lord Mayor, three justices, eight members of the jury and more than 40 other people who had been present. All the victims were said to have been sitting on the left hand side of the court.

During the eighteenth century, the incidence of tuberculosis increased markedly because thousands of people were deprived of air and light by the introduction of the Window Tax in 1696. This encouraged landlords to brick up windows in the properties they owned in order to reduce their liability for the new tax, but the health of those living and working in these buildings inevitably suffered.

The greatest contribution to preventive medicine at this time was the discovery of a vaccine against smallpox, which had been widespread in Britain from the seventeenth century onwards, with many severe epidemics (Baldry, 1976). Limited immunity obtained from sniffing the powdered, dry crust of smallpox pustules had

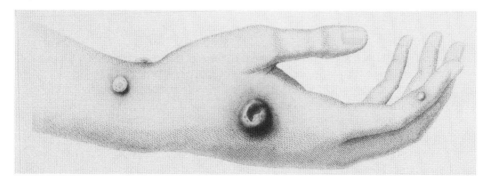

Fig 1.4   The hand of Sarah Nelmes
(Reproduced by kind permission of the Wellcome Institute Library, London)

been recorded in China from the eleventh century, but it was not until 1718 that Lady Mary Wortley Montague, wife of the British Ambassador in Turkey, introduced the Eastern practice of inoculation into England. The method used was to induce a mild form of the disease by drawing a thread soaked in fluid from a smallpox pustule through a small incision made in the arm (Baldry, 1965, 1976). King George I allowed experimental inoculations to be carried out on six prisoners at Newgate Gaol who had been condemned to death. The men were told that if they survived they would be pardoned. They all lived and the agreement was honoured (Williams, 1975).

Edward Jenner (1749–1823), a Gloucestershire physician, demonstrated that immunity to smallpox had been conferred on an eight-year-old boy whom he 'vaccinated' with pus from blisters on the hands of the dairymaid, Sarah Nelmes, suffering from cowpox (figure 1.4). Thus, this preventive technique derived its name from the Latin word for cow – 'vacca'.

THE NINETEENTH CENTURY

At the beginning of the nineteenth century infectious diseases were rife. The three most prevalent in the UK were smallpox, tuberculosis and cholera.

Vaccination against smallpox became compulsory in England in 1853 following an epidemic which killed 41 000 people.

Tuberculosis was popularly known as 'the captain of death'. The Industrial Revolution, with its atmospheric pollution and overcrowding in the cities, brought social changes tailormade for the spread of pulmonary tuberculosis, or 'consumption' as it was known, although, by the end of the century, an awareness emerged that the disease might be successfully treated by judicious diet, fresh air and rest.

An epidemic of cholera in 1832 decimated the UK population, 1 in every 131 people dying. The clothes and possessions of the dead were ordered to be burned or buried in quicklime. The poor frequently rioted against such enforced precautions, so many of the dead were buried at night. In filthy, crowded, insanitary social conditions the disease became known as 'King Cholera' (figure 1.5).

Doctors tried various remedies: cold water and ice, hot compresses and baths, hot air to warm a patient's bed (although one patient's bed was set on fire), the application of electricity which unfortunately killed one patient, bleeding, the wearing of a flannel collar or belt around the stomach, and the drinking of sea water.

This epidemic obliged the authorities to consider public health. A civil servant, Edwin Chadwick, showed that the average age at death was 43 years for gentlemen, 30 for tradesmen and 22 for labourers. He concluded that disease was spread by atmospheric pollution caused by overcrowding, poor water supplies, bad drainage and dirty towns. His initiative to clean streets, improve the quality of water supplies and provide sewage disposal facilities were incorporated into a Public Health Act in 1848.

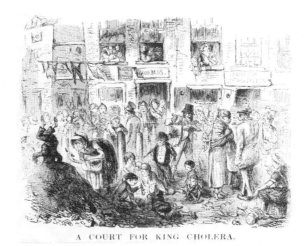

A COURT FOR KING CHOLERA.

Fig 1.5   'A court for King Cholera' is hardly an exaggeration of many dwelling-places of the very poor
in London
(Reproduced by kind permission of the Wellcome Institute Library, London)

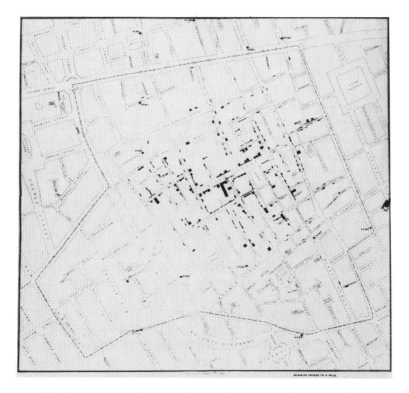

Fig 1.6   A map showing deaths from cholera in the Golden Square district
(Reproduced by kind permission of the Wellcome Institute Library, London)

In the summer of 1854, a cholera outbreak in Golden Square, London, resulted in approximately 500 deaths (figure 1.6). During the outbreak John Snow (1813–1858), a London doctor, observed that, because the pump in Broad Street had a reputation for particularly good water, the people came from some distance to use it (Winterton, 1980). Dr Snow postulated that the well must be the source of the trouble, having been contaminated by the evacuations of someone living nearby. A later investigation showed that the brick lining of a cesspool about 3 ft away was cracked and decayed, and it is probable that this was responsible for contaminating the previously drinkable water.

The view held at that time was that the cholera 'poison' was airborne and, therefore, impossible to eradicate. Dr Snow argued that the symptoms of diarrhoea and vomiting must be caused by direct contact of the bacillus with the alimentary canal. He persuaded the authorities to remove the handle of the water pump, the outbreak subsided, and Dr Snow proved that cholera was a waterborne infection.

During the epidemic, many patients were nursed at the nearby Middlesex Hospital, which, at that time, had 200 beds. Considering that 120 cases of cholera were admitted in three days, the incidence of cross-infection was remarkably low. Only two nurses, one laundry worker and one patient became infected, and all except one of the nurses recovered. The normal complement of nurses for each 20-bed ward was one sister and one nurse by day, and one or no nurse by night but, during the outbreak, extra nurses were employed, among whom was Florence Nightingale.

Microbiology as a Science

The nineteenth century saw the revival of medicine as a scientific discipline. The idea that an infection might be caused by the unseen entry into the body of a tiny, invisible organism had first been recorded by the Roman encyclopaedist Varro one hundred years before the birth of Christ. In 1685, Francisco Redi attempted to refute the then-accepted theory of spontaneous generation by asserting that only life can produce life (Williams, 1981).

This theory was finally laid to rest by Louis Pasteur (1822–1895), a French chemist, who proved that living organisms arise only from exactly similar living organisms.

Pasteur's work involved him in the study of fermentation processes. He showed that, whereas fermentation of beer and wines was brought about by yeasts, that of butyric and lactic acids was accomplished by bacteria. Pasteur postulated, and then demonstrated, that these organisms could be destroyed by heat treatment of equipment, dressings and water and devised many techniques for growing and identifying organisms which are the basis of those used today.

Pasteur also identified the means of spread of anthrax, cholera and rabies and, through his discovery that immunity could be afforded by inoculation with a weakened culture of a microorganism, went on to produce vaccines against these diseases.

The scientific study of microbiology was taken a step further by Robert Koch

(1843–1910), a German general practitioner, who, after receiving a second-hand microscope as a birthday present, continued Pasteur's investigations into *Mycobacterium tuberculosis*, *Vibrio cholerae* and *Bacillus anthracis* (Coleman, 1985). Koch's paper, 'The Etiology of Traumatic Infective Diseases', first published in 1879, proved the microbial theory of disease beyond a shadow of a doubt. Koch cultured the anthrax bacillus and reproduced the disease in animals by injecting them with his cultures.

Koch and his assistants also established a systematic classification of bacteria and introduced the use of aniline dyes for staining, solid-agar growth media and oil-immersion microscope lenses.

Microbiology in Practice

Long before these advances in identifying organisms were made, the methods of spread of many infections had been appreciated if not acknowledged. Accounts of puerperal or 'child-bed' fever were recorded thousands of years before mortality figures from the new Westminster lying-in hospital were announced. At this hospital, between 13 November 1769 and 15 May 1770, 19 out of 65 women delivered became infected, and 14 died (Williams, 1975). Suggestions that there were too many beds and that the wards were poorly ventilated went unheeded.

Later, around 1790, Alexander Hamilton, Professor of Midwifery at Edinburgh University, noted the link between erysipelas and puerperal fever. The causative organism of both conditions has now been shown to the beta-haemolytic Lancefield group A streptococcus.

The American Oliver Holmes, in 1843, made himself unpopular when he associated maternal death with midwives' dirty hands. Then, in 1847, Ignaz Zemmelweiss, a Hungarian doctor, conducted what is probably the most important hand-washing research of all time. Of the two obstetric clinics in his hospital, he recorded a higher death rate from puerperal fever in the clinic attended by medical students than in that attended by midwives. He observed that the medical students, on leaving the dissecting room, would proceed to perform vaginal examinations and deliveries without washing their hands. He observed that the midwives did not perform dissections and did wash their hands.

Zemmelweiss then proceeded to instruct the medical students coming from the post-mortem room to wash their hands in chloride of lime. Two years later, the maternal death rate had been reduced by 90 per cent. Ahead of their time, his explanations were poorly received, and in 1861 he was admitted to a mental hospital where he died of an infection that he had contracted while he was operating.

The principles of asepsis were now gradually being introduced into operating theatres. Previously, surgeons had operated in old, blood-stained frockcoats with ligatures threaded through their buttonholes; instruments were unsterilised, hands were not washed before operating and dirty bandages were used as many times as possible.

Professor Joseph Lister (1827–1912), in Glasgow, began to question why the evils of 'hospitalism' – gangrene, erysipelas and pyaemia – were encountered more frequently in hospitals than in private houses. Lister followed on from Pasteur's work on fermentation by suggesting that the putrefaction of proteins leading to pus formation might be caused by a similar process also involving bacteria. Previously, it had been believed that 'laudable pus' was always necessary for a patient's recovery, whereas now it was proposed that pus might indicate the presence of disease.

In 1867, Lister devised a spray which pumped carbolic acid into the operating area, killing the bacteria around. Hence, the start of each operation was accompanied by the chant, 'Let us spray'. Carbolic putty was similarly applied to compound fractures in an attempt to prevent gangrene.

In 1886, the first operation performed under sterile conditions was undertaken in Germany (Hastings, 1974). In 1890, William Stewart Halstead pioneered the use of rubber surgical gloves, and in 1889 gauze face-masks were introduced, both aiming to limit the spread of infection.

TROPICAL DISEASE

At the turn of the nineteenth century, sleeping sickness was epidemic in Africa, and malaria and yellow fever were endemic. In the early twentieth century, Sir David Bruce showed that sleeping sickness was due to a parasite carried by the tsetse fly (Williams, 1981). The spread of disease was limited by the destruction of flies and their breeding grounds and by restricting the movement of infected people.

The first proof that malaria was transmitted by the mosquito was furnished by Sir Patrick Manson, medical officer in Formosa, whose 1879 paper on the subject was met with disbelief. However, the Indian army doctor Ronald Ross and Giovanni Grassi from Rome substantiated these facts at the end of the nineteenth century.

Yellow fever was, in 1898, rampant in Cuba. Two investigating doctors allowed themselves to be bitten by infected mosquitoes; one man died, the other recovered, and the connection between mosquitoes and yellow fever was established. To demonstrate that the fever was not contagious if mosquitoes were absent, volunteers slept over a period of three weeks in the soiled bedding of yellow fever victims. None of these volunteers became infected. The chain of infection had been broken by isolating victims, both suspected and proven, from mosquitoes.

The Panama Canal, vitally important for world trade, would not have been completed if malaria and yellow fever had not been controlled. Workers on the canal in 1888 were dying from these diseases at a rate of 176 per 1000. When the canal was finished in 1914, the death rate had reduced to only 6 per 1000 men.

MICROBIOLOGY AND MAN

Infectious disease has been a deadlier enemy to mankind than has war:

● 'Of some 300 000 crusaders who left Western Europe in 1096 only 20 000

Table 1.1   Events in the modern era of infectious disease

19th century	Separation of waste water and drinking water by construction of sewers and water supply systems reduces the levels of many infectious diseases
1854	Cholera epidemiology discovered by John Snow
1850–80	The birth of true microbiology. The existence, occurrence and role of bacteria and viruses in infectious disease was elucidated by Louis Pasteur, Robert Koch, Ignaz Zemmelweiss, Joseph Lister and many others
1904	Salvarsan, the first true antimicrobial drug, produced by Paul Ehrlich
1906	The first useful diagnostic serology test carried out by August Wasserman for detecting syphilis infection
1934	Development of chloroquine, an anti-malarial drug
1935	Prontos 1, the first sulphonamide, discovered by Gerhard Danagk
1939	DDT discovered by Paul Muller, enabling insect-borne diseases (typhus, malaria, yellow fever, etc.) to be controlled
1940	First purification of penicillin by Howard Florey and Ernst Chain after an original observation by Alexander Fleming in 1928
1946	Mosquitoes start to become resistant to DDT
1944–50	Era of discovery of the other early antibiotics – streptomycin (1944), chloramphenicol (1947) and cephalosporin (1948)
1959	The first evidence of transferrable antibiotic resistance emerges
1961	First reports of chloroquine-resistant malaria
1980	Global eradication of wild smallpox announced by the World Health Organisation
1980s	Genetic engineering and monoclonal antibodies had their initial impact on health care
1980s	Emergence of human immune deficiency virus linked with acquired immunodeficiency syndrome

reached the Holy City [Jerusalem]. Bubonic plague destroyed a third of the people in medieval Europe. Imported smallpox beginning in the West Indies where Columbus landed wiped out whole tribes of American Indians. Christianity flourished as the Indians found their Gods powerless to halt death and destruction. The Indians, however, had their revenge and with Columbus' return sent syphilis to Europe. The ruin of Bonaparte's Moscow campaign was completed by typhus which killed 300 000 French soldiers in the Peninsular war. In the Crimean war cholera, smallpox and typhus killed ten times as many British soldiers as were killed in action. Typhus alone was responsible for the deaths of nearly a million soldiers. The first time that more men died in battle than from disease was in the Franco–Prussian war (1870–1871).' (Hastings, 1974)

An understanding of microbiology has been a long time in coming (table 1.1). Progress in acquiring medical knowledge has been hindered by social and religious beliefs and pressures, and microbiology has emerged as a comparatively new science. It will continue to evolve and health-care workers need to keep abreast of developments. History has shown what happens when knowledge is lacking or minds are closed. Valid health care today requires that science and informed activity supersede custom and practice. Microorganisms develop in response to the environment and to changes in therapeutic regimes. Health-care workers need to be constantly vigilant: microbiology is a dynamic science.

References

Baldry P (1976) *The Battle Against Bacteria: A Fresh Look*. Cambridge: Cambridge University Press.

Coleman V (1985) *The Story of Medicine*. London: Robert Hale.

Hastings R P (1974) *Medicine and International History*. London: Ernest Benn.

McGrew R (1985) *Encyclopaedia of Medical History*. London: Macmillan.

Williams G (1981) *The Age of Miracles; Medicine and Surgery in the Nineteenth Century*. London: Constable.

Zeigler P (1969) *The Black Death*. London: Collins.

Further Reading

Baly M E (1980) *Nursing and Social Change*, 2nd edn. London: Heinemann Medical.

Bibbings J M (1986) The history of wound dressings. *Nursing*, 3(5):169–173.

Galbraith N S (1984) Medicine International. *Investigation and Control of an Acute Episode of Disease*, pp. 1–7.

Gordon R (1983) *Great Medical Disasters*. London: Hutchinson.

Horton R (1985) Disinfection through the ages. *Nursing Times, Journal of Infection Control Nursing*, pp. 17–19.

Klebs A C (1917) The history of infection. *Annals of Medical History*, 1917, pp. 159–173.

Roper N (1982) *Principles of Nursing*, 3rd edn. Edinburgh: Churchill Livingstone.

Williams G (1975) *The Age of Agony, the Art of Healing, circa 1700–1800*. London: Constable.

Winterton W R (1980) The Soho cholera epidemic, 1854. *History of Medicine*, 8(11): 11–20.

Worsley M A (1983) *Guidance for Hospital Personnel. Control of Hospital Acquired Infections*. London: Update.

2

Microorganisms and their

Properties

The aim of this chapter is to outline the basic properties and characteristics of microorganisms. A knowledge of their characteristic behaviour patterns will allow health-care workers to identify the microorganisms' mode of spread and use this as a basis for planning appropriate, individualised care while, at the same time, preventing cross-infection.

The term microorganism, or microbe, is used to describe any plant or animal which is too small to be seen with the naked eye. Microorganisms are classified in order of decreasing complexity: algae, fungi, protozoa, bacteria, mycoplasma, rickettsia, chlamydia and viruses (Blackwell and Weir, 1981). Microbes are usually single-celled although the fungi can be considerably more complex.

The microbial world is extensive as nature endeavours to populate every conceivable space with organisms. Microorganisms will be found nearly every-where where active steps have not been taken to remove them. They are ubiquitous in the soil, in hot springs, in the sea, high in the air, in vegetable matter, on animals and in dust. The type of microbial life present will be determined by the available food-stuffs and the prevailing physical conditions. One would not, for example, see the blue–green mould that appears on a stale crust of bread growing in an open wound.

Many organisms live independently of man and those that are dependent exist in a host–organism relationship that is generally harmless and may be mutually beneficial. Of the vast array of organisms, only about 50 or so species are, in fact, pathogenically disposed towards humans. When they invade and damage the human host, these organisms run the gauntlet of being destroyed, either in the initial immune response or on the resulting death of the host.

THE RELATIONSHIP BETWEEN HOST AND MICROORGANISM

Microorganisms are part of the ecological chain (figure 2.1). In this chain all the participants can be grouped in accordance with what they do. First are the producers, the green plants, which convert inorganic material into organic by using the energy of the sun. Second are the consumers: man and other animals who obtain their energy by feeding on plants or each other. The third group comprises

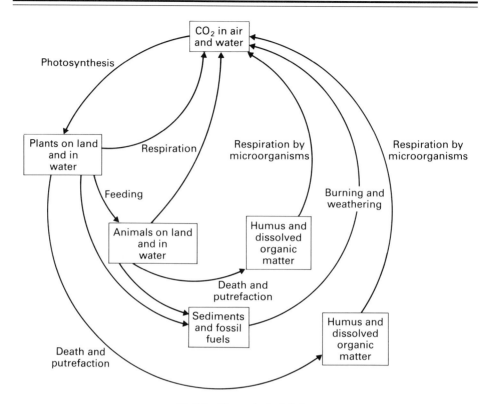

Fig 2.1   The ecological chain

the fungi and bacteria which decompose dead plants and animals and return their component substances to the soil where they are in turn used by the plants. Advertisers encourage us to buy disinfectants and literally pour them down the drain to eliminate 'all known germs'; fortunately the effect of such disinfectants on the total microbial population, necessary to perpetuate the ecological cycle, is negligible.

Despite the fact that man is composed of millions of cells, whereas a microorganism is a single cell, it is a continual battle for man to retain the upper hand in the host–organism relationship. Man belongs to a group that are **eukaryotic** or complicated in cell structure. The majority of microbes are **prokaryotic** or of simple cell structure (table 2.1). Both eukaryotic and prokaryotic organisms are concerned with the survival of their own species through growth and reproduction. Survival is achieved in the single microbial cell and in all the millions of mammalian cells by:

1. *Catabolic processes*   Organic material is broken down to release energy for the cell's use.

2. *Anabolic processes*   Energy is used to build structural and functional components of the cell.

3. *Reproductive processes*   The genetic material of the cell is contained within the nucleus as giant molecules (macromolecules) of **deoxyribonucleic acid (DNA).**

Table 2.1   Eukaryotic and prokaryotic organisms

Eukaryotic (complex structure)	Prokaryotic (simple structure)
Multicellular with extensive differentiation Vertebrates Invertebrates Seed plants Ferns Mosses and liverworts *Multicellular without differentiation, or unicellular* Algae Fungi Protozoa	*Unicellar* Bacteria Mycoplasma Rickettsia Chlamydia Viruses

Ribonucleic acid (RNA) is another macromolecule and is present in the cell's cytoplasm. The information coded for by DNA is **translated** by RNA into specific proteins which form the structural and functional components of the cell (figure 2.2).

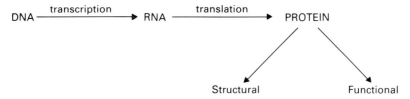

Fig 2.2   Protein synthesis

If a microorganism lacks any of the necessary components for these three processes, the situation may be rectified by obtaining the necessary materials from the host's cells. For example, although chlamydia contain DNA and RNA, they do not possess any energy-yielding processes so rely on the host cell to supply energy-rich compounds. Viruses are even more dependent on the host as they contain only one type of nucleic acid – either DNA or RNA. Generally, the more specialised a microbe becomes for a parasitic existence, the more infectious is the disease which it causes.

THE EUKARYOTIC CELL

The mammalian cell illustrated in figure 2.3 is a typical eukaryotic cell. The **nucleus** has a distinct structure inside the cytoplasm of the cell. It is surrounded by a **nuclear membrane** and contains DNA, the genetic material of the cell, in the form of **chromosomes**. When the cell divides each chromosome is replicated and a complete set is passed to each daughter cell by **mitosis** (figure 2.4). A number of other

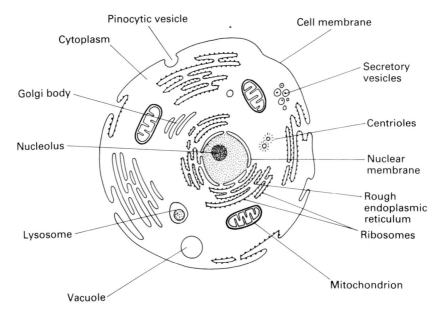

Fig 2.3   A eukaryotic cell as seen under the electron microscope

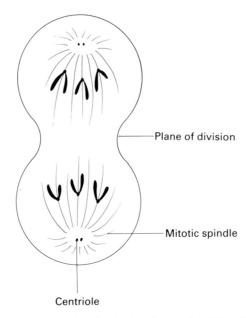

Fig 2.4   Mitosis. The nuclear envelope has broken down and the DNA, having replicated, has condensed into two sets of chromosomes. One set is distributed to each of the two new daughter cells by a mitotic spindle

definitive structures (**organelles**) are observed within the cell:

- *Nucleolus*: concerned with the production, within the nucleus, of RNA
- *Ribosomes*: where proteins are produced
- *Rough endoplasmic reticulum*: concerned with the transport of substances around the cell
- *Golgi body*: substances to be secreted from the cell are assembled here
- *Pinocytic vesicles*: some substances are taken into the cell in these organelles
- *Lysosomes*: contain the enzyme lysozyme which is able to destroy unwanted organelles
- *Secretory vesicles*: contain substances produced within the cell
- *Mitochondrion*: the site of internal respiration
- *Centrosomes*: concerned with spindle formation during mitosis

Eukaryotic Microorganisms

Algae

Algae are single-celled green plants and are not of any medical significance.

Fungi

The fungi include the yeasts and moulds and are described in detail by Thomas (1979). Unlike algae, fungi do not possess chlorophyll but feed on living plants and animals and decaying organic matter. Fungal infections in humans are called **mycoses** and are classified as:

1. *Systemic or deep mycoses* involving internal organs, especially the lungs, e.g. histoplasmosis infection.
2. *Subcutaneous or superficial mycoses* which grow in the deeper layers of the skin or outer layers of hair, skin and nails, e.g. athlete's foot, ringworm, thrush (candida) infections.

When considering man's competition with microorganisms, fungi are particularly interesting. Many antibiotics produced to combat bacterial infections are derived from fungi. While this has been generally beneficial there has, in recent years, been an increase in the frequency of fungal infections as a direct result of the widespread use of antibiotics. These antibiotics destroy the normal bacterial flora of the mucosa, allowing the fungal 'weeds' to flourish and grow without competition.

Protozoa

Protozoa are single-celled organisms which mostly spend their time feeding on dead organic matter in the environment. There are a few that cause disease in man: *Plasmodium* species (causing malaria), *Trypanosoma* species (leading to African sleeping sickness) and *Entamoeba* species (giving rise to amoebic dysentery).

THE PROKARYOTIC CELL

The bacterium illustrated in figure 2.5 is an example of a prokaryotic cell. There is no membrane-bound nucleus, no endoplasmic reticulum, mitochrondria or Golgi body. The **mesosome**, formed by unfolding of the cell membrane, is the site of cell respiration and is functionally equivalent to the mitochondria of eukaryotic cells. The cytoplasm does contain ribosomes, enzymes and storage granules, but in a less organised form than in eukaryotic cells. The shape of the bacterium is maintained by a rigid **cell wall** which is not found surrounding eukaryotic cells. Outside the cell wall there may be additional layers of material and a protective coat or **capsule** may surround the bacterial cell. As there is only one chromosome, mitosis does not take place; reproduction is by **binary fission**. When the cell divides the DNA replicates and the daughter chromosomes are drawn apart (figure 2.6).

Prokaryotic cells are much simpler than eukaryotic cells but can still contain all the components necessary for an independent existence.

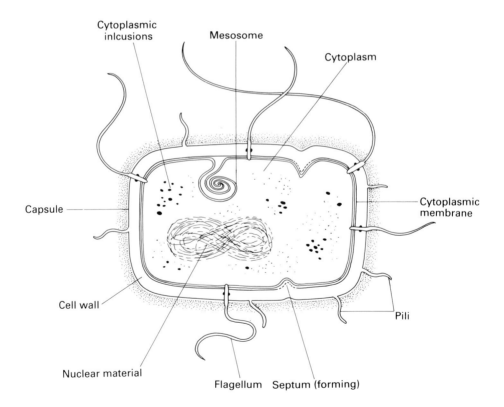

Fig 2.5   Diagram of a typical prokaryotic bacterial cell

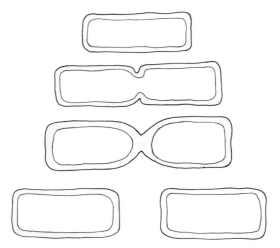

Fig 2.6   Binary fission. The bacterial cell elongates and, as the cell wall grows across the cell, divides to two smaller cells which then grow and multiply in turn

Prokaryotic Microorganisms: Bacteria

Bacteria are microscopically small organisms. They are measured in microns (μ, i.e. 0.001 mm) and range from 0.3 to 14 μ in length. Three hundred of the smaller organisms could be placed end to end across the diameter of a pin head and, therefore, a microscope is needed to observe them.

Bacteria are classified according to three main properties:

1. Gram stain
2. Shape (morphology)
3. Oxygen requirement

Gram Staining

In their natural state when viewed under the microscope, bacteria are seen as tiny, colourless organisms. To make them more identifiable they can be stained with a dye, usually methylene blue. Gram-positive organisms retain this dye following decolourising treatment with acetone, and appear a deep violet colour under the microscope. Gram-negative organisms, however, lose the violet stain in the decolourisation process but take up a red counter-stain and appear pink.

Staphylococcus aureus, which causes skin infections, is a typical Gram-positive organism (figure 2.7). *Escherichia coli*, part of the normal flora of the bowel and a common cause of urinary tract infection, is a typical Gram-negative organism (figure 2.8).

The mycobacterium group of organisms, e.g. *Mycobacterium tuberculosis*, are not readily seen by the Gram-stain method. These bacilli have abundant lipids in their cell wall which makes chemical penetration by the Gram stain difficult, so are

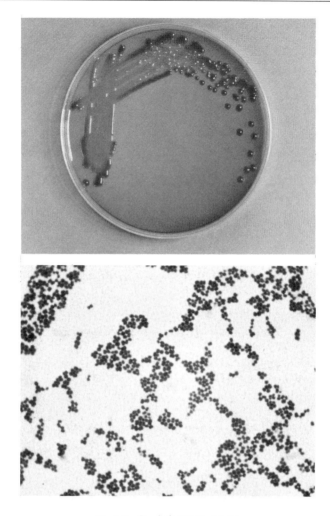

Fig 2.7 *Staphylococcus aureus*

examined by an acid-fast or Ziehl–Nielsen stain, hence the terms 'acid-fast bacilli' (AFB) and 'Ziehl–Nielsen (ZN) positive' which are used to describe them.

Morphology

Bacteria are classified into four main groups by their shape:

1. *Cocci* which are round
2. *Bacilli* which are rod-shaped
3. *Coccobacilli* which are very short rods and may resemble cocci
4. *Spirochaetes* which are spiral

Bacteria can be grown in a nutrient broth or culture medium. In this laboratory setting the manner in which these bacteria arrange themselves can be observed

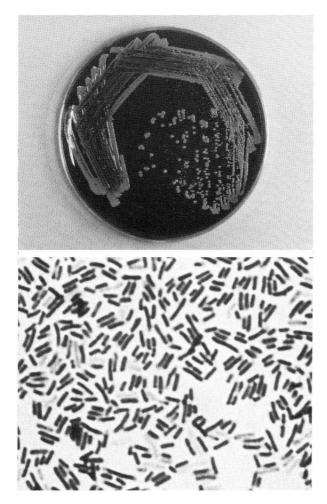

Fig 2.8 *Escherichia coli*

(figure 2.9). Some grow in chains (**streptococci**), some in pairs (**diplococci**) and some in clusters (**staphylococci**).

An alternative shape sometimes observed is that of the spore. Under adverse conditions two groups of Gram-positive bacteria, the genera *Bacillus* and *Clostridium*, produce structures called **endospores**, commonly referred to as spores. In the case of *Clostridium* (figure 2.10) they are produced singly within the cell. A mature spore can survive in a dormant state in dust, vegetation or soil, for weeks, months or even years, until it eventually finds itself in an environment suitable for its germination (figure 2.11). As a spore the organism will be considerably more resistant to heat, cold and disinfectants than was the original bacterium. This may cause additional problems in the hospital environment, for instance in the sterilisation of theatre instruments.

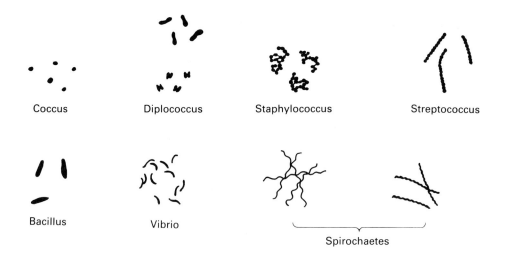

Fig 2.9   Morphology of bacteria

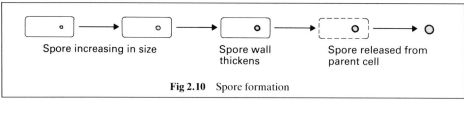

Fig 2.10   Spore formation

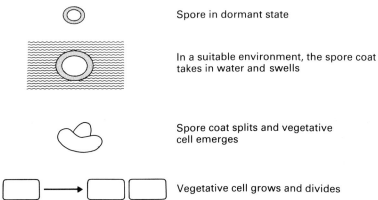

Spore in dormant state

In a suitable environment, the spore coat takes in water and swells

Spore coat splits and vegetative cell emerges

Vegetative cell grows and divides

Fig 2.11   Spore germination

Oxygen Requirement

Some bacteria must have oxygen in their environment in order to grow. These are classified as **obligate aerobes**. Others cannot tolerate the presence of oxygen and these are classified as **obligate anaerobes**. Some, **facultative anaerobes**, are able to grow with or without oxygen.

A summary of the classification of medically important bacteria according to Gram stain, shape and oxygen requirement is given in tables 2.2 and 2.3.

Table 2.2 Classification of medically important Gram-positive bacteria

	Oxygen requirement	Growth pattern	Genus/species example
Cocci	Aerobes or facultative anaerobes	Clusters	Staphylococcus/*Staph. aureus*
		Chains or pairs	Streptococcus/*Strep. pyogenes*
	Anaerobes	Chains or pairs	Streptococcus/*Strep. putridus*
Bacilli	Aerobes or facultative anaerobes	Sporing	Bacillus/*B. anthracis*
		Non-sporing	Corynebacterium/*C. diphtheriae*
	Anaerobes	Sporing	Clostridium/*Cl. tetani*
		Non-sporing	Actinomycetes/*A. israelii*

Differences Between Gram-Positive and Gram-Negative Bacteria

The Gram stain is useful as it can distinguish structural differences between, and help to give an understanding of the disease-causing capabilities of, Gram-positive and Gram-negative bacteria. Structural differences between the two are illustrated in figure 2.12. Note that the Gram-negative bacteria have a space between the cytoplasmic membrane and the mucopeptide layer, the **periplasmic space**, in which a number of enzymes are found. The Gram-positive bacteria have a much thicker cell wall (**mucopeptide layer**) than do Gram-negative ones. Outside the cell wall Gram-negative bacteria have a layer of **lipopolysaccharide** (LPS) which is a complex of sugars, fatty acids and phosphate, whereas Gram-positive bacteria have a layer of **teichoic acid** which is a complex of sugar and phosphate.

Both types of bacteria may be enclosed in a **capsule**. This is a layer of gelatinous material produced by the bacterium itself which adheres to the outside of the cell and shields the bacterium from host defence mechanisms.

An important structure seen in Gram-negative bacteria and in some Gram-positive bacilli is the **flagellum** (plural flagella). This is a whip-like appendage which originates from inside the cell membrane. Flagella may be present in groups or singly and are capable of inducing movement in the bacterium. Thus, generally, Gram-negative bacteria are motile while Gram-positive organisms (apart from some Gram-positive bacilli) are non-motile. This has important consequences when the routes of bacterial spread are examined (see later chapters). If both groups are examined under a microscope, Gram-negative bacteria are observed to move or 'swim', while Gram-positive cocci move only by Brownian movement which leads to a rapid oscillation of each bacterium within a very limited area due to its

Table 2.3   Classification of medically important Gram-negative bacteria

	Oxygen requirement	Genus/species example
Cocci	Aerobes or facultative anaerobes	Neisseria/*N. meningitidis, N. gonorrhoeae*
	Anaerobes	Veillonella/*V. parvula*
Bacilli	Aerobes or facultative anaerobes	Pseudomonas/*Pseud.aeruginosa*
		Enterobacteria: Salmonella/*Salm. typhi* Shigella/*Sh. sonnei* Klebsiella/*Klebs. aerogenes* Proteus/*P. mirabilis* Escherichia/*E. coli* Serratia/*S. marcescens*
		Parvobacteria: Yersinia/*Y. pestis* Bordetella/*Bord. pertussis* Haemophilus/*H. influenzae* Brucella/*B. abortus*
		Vibrios: Campylobacter/*C. jejuni* Vibrio/*V. cholerae*
		Legionella/*L. pneumophila*
	Anaerobes	Bacteroides/*B. fragilis*
Spirochaetes	Aerobes	Leptospira/*L. interrogans*
	Anaerobes	Borrelia/*Borrelia vincentii* Treponema/*Trep. pallidum*

bombardment by water molecules. This property means that Gram-negative bacteria tend to spread by a 'wet' route and Gram-positive via a 'dry' one.

Bacterial Growth and Reproduction

As mentioned above, bacteria reproduce by a process known as binary fission. This is a simple process by which one cell divides into two parts. While the parent bacterial cell elongates by growing the genetic material, one circular double strand of DNA replicates itself and segregates between two parts of the cell. Cell walls then grow across the bacterium to separate the two daughter cells thus formed. Each of these daughter cells will grow and later divide. The rate of growth or the time it takes a cell or population to divide varies between different types of bacteria; some such as *Escherichia coli* divide every 20 minutes so, under ideal conditions, a single organism can multiply to give 512 daughter cells in three hours or a million in under eight hours. Others, such as *Mycobacterium tuberculosis*, are very slow growers. It is, therefore, not surprising that laboratory reports showing a

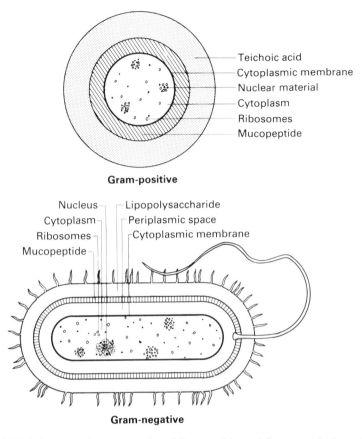

Gram-positive

Teichoic acid
Cytoplasmic membrane
Nuclear material
Cytoplasm
Ribosomes
Mucopeptide

Nucleus — Lipopolysaccharide
Cytoplasm — Periplasmic space
Ribosomes — Cytoplasmic membrane
Mucopeptide

Gram-negative

Fig 2.12 Diagrammatic representation of Gram-positive and Gram-negative bacteria

growth of *E. coli* in a urine specimen can be returned to the ward the next day, whereas it might be three or more weeks before *M. tuberculosis* can be grown and identified.

The rapid growth of some organisms can cause considerable infection control hazards. A famous example of this was the Bundaberg tragedy, which occurred in Australia in 1928 not long after the introduction of diptheria inoculations (Andrews, 1976). Twenty-nine children were injected with the diptheria anti-toxin. Within 12 hours 18 children were ill and, before two days passed, 12 children had died. The facts about this horrific incident soon emerged. The single, rubber-capped bottle of mixture had originally been sterile, but had been used the week before to successfully inoculate a number of children. Before each injection a hypodermic needle was pushed through the rubber cap to draw up the anti-toxin. This needle must have picked up a few *Staphylococcus aureus* organisms from the skin of the first group of children and transplanted them into the supposedly sterile bottle. During the bottle's week on the shelf the staphylococci would have multiplied to many millions. This highly contaminated solution was then injected into the second group of children the following week, resulting in a fatal septicaemia in some.

Bacterial Genetics

In addition to the deoxyribonucleic acid (DNA) of the chromosome, bacteria may have small, circular units of DNA in the cytoplasm which are known as **plasmids**. This extra DNA is not required for growth or replication and so can be lost or acquired without harming the cell. It is particularly important in the acquisition of antibiotic resistance by bacterial cells, and one plasmid may code for resistance to several antibiotics.

Bacteria exist in a dynamic relationship with the environment to which they constantly adapt and respond. Response to selective pressures may result in gradual mutation of the bacterial chromosome. For example, the use of an antibiotic will select out mutated cells that are antibiotic-resistant. This is a slow process but is significant when patients are on long-term antibiotic therapy, such as that for tuberculosis. In such cases, several antibiotics are given simultaneously to prevent such selection.

Transfer of genetic material can occur from one cell to another in three ways:

1. Transformation
2. Transduction
3. Conjugation

Transformation   In this process DNA lying free of its parent bacterial cell is taken up into another bacterial cell and incorporated into its chromosome (figure 2.13). The DNA must be from a closely related strain with adequate homology. This DNA may confer a new property such as antibiotic resistance. Transformation is not a very efficient method of promoting bacterial adaptability.

Transduction   DNA from the nucleus or cytoplasm can be transferred from one cell to another by a bacterial virus known as a **bacteriophage**. As the DNA all has to be packaged into the viral head, the amount that can be transferred is limited, but this method provides the main method of transfer of resistance among *Staphylococcus aureus* organisms in hospitals and is, therefore, of particular importance (figure 2.14, p. 32).

Conjugation   Conjugation is an important means of genetic transfer, particularly of antibiotic resistance, for Gram-negative bacteria (figure 2.15, p. 33). For this process to occur the sex pilus of one donor or 'male' cell must attach to the sex pilus of another sensitive recipient or 'female' cell. Plasmid replication occurs; one copy of the plasmid is transferred to the sensitive cell and the other copy remains in the original cell. Information for formation of the sex pilus and for replication and transfer of the plasmid is coded for by the DNA of the plasmid. Unlike transduction, there is no limitation to the amount of genetic material which can be transferred by the plasmid in conjugation.

Widespread and indiscriminate use of antibiotics can result in rapid bacterial

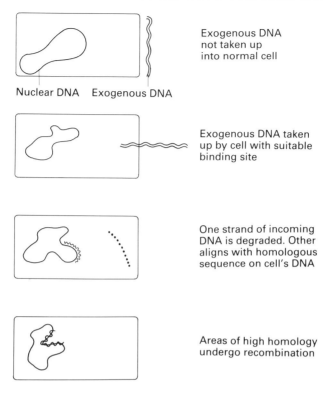

Exogenous DNA
not taken up
into normal cell

Nuclear DNA   Exogenous DNA

Exogenous DNA taken
up by cell with suitable
binding site

One strand of incoming
DNA is degraded. Other
aligns with homologous
sequence on cell's DNA

Areas of high homology
undergo recombination

Fig 2.13   Transformation

resistance by any combination of the processes described above. For this reason, hospitals should have clear antibiotic control policies (see chapter 7).

COMMON INFECTIVE ORGANISMS

The organisms discussed below are those commonly encountered in hospitals (see tables 2.2 and 2.3 above).

Gram-Positive Cocci

Staphylococci

Staphylococcus aureus is an important skin pathogen which is responsible for both superficial and deep infections, e.g. boils, impetigo and surgical wound infections. It is also responsible for certain toxin-mediated diseases such as the scalded skin syndrome, toxic shock syndrome and staphylococcal food poisoning. *Staph. aureus* is found in the anterior nares of the nose in approximately 20–30 per cent of healthy people.

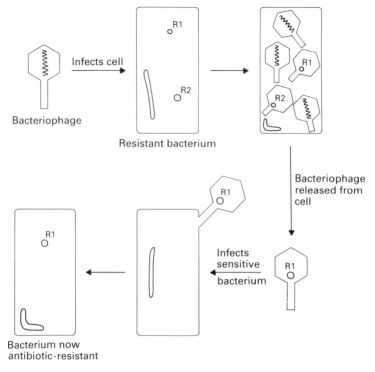

Fig 2.14 Transduction

Another staphylococcal species, *Staph. epidermidis*, is present as part of the normal skin flora and rarely causes infections, although it may cause serious problems at the sites of prostheses and central venous lines.

These two staphylococcal species are distinguished by their ability to clot plasma by means of the enzyme coagulase. *Staph. aureus* is **coagulase positive** (i.e. has the ability to clot plasma) whereas *Staph. epidermidis* is **coagulase negative**.

Streptococci

Streptococci may inhabit the mucous membranes of man and animals, including those of the mouth, upper respiratory tract and intestine. Some streptococci live in food, especially milk and dairy products, where they are found with the lactobacillus. Those that discolour or destroy red blood cells are called **haemolytic streptococci**. They can be identified on a growth medium (**blood agar**) which contains red blood cells.

Bacteria that produce complete **lysis**, i.e. destruction of blood cells, on blood agar have a clear area around the bacterial colony and are called **beta-(β–) haemolytic streptococci**. They are the commonest cause of streptococcal infections and are classified into Lancefield groups A to S.

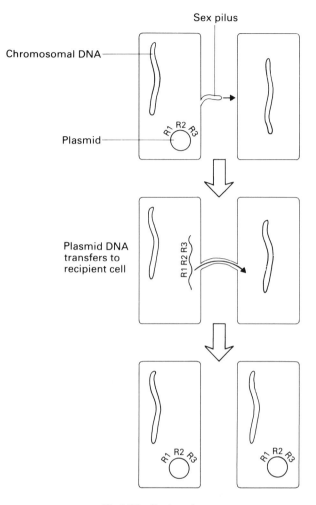

Fig 2.15 Conjugation

The beta-haemolytic streptococcus of Lancefield group A (*Strep. pyogenes*) is probably the most important human pathogen in this group. The disease produced is often determined by the portal of entry of the organism. *Strep. pyogenes* causes infections of the throat and skin, such as erysipelas, or puerperal sepsis following childbirth. It also produces a toxin that results in the systemic body rash of scarlet fever.

Lancefield group B streptococci can cause infections in neonates if the organism is acquired from the mother's vagina during delivery. Approximately 30 per cent of all women have group B streptococci present in their normal vaginal flora.

Alpha–(α–)haemolytic streptococci, e.g. *Strep. viridans*, produce incomplete lysis of red cells which appears as a greenish colour change around the colony on blood agar. *Strep. viridans* are present as normal oral flora but can cause subacute bacterial endocarditis in patients with already damaged heart valves if they enter the blood stream after, for instance, dental surgery.

Non-haemolytic streptococci are usually harmless but are very occasionally pathogenic. *Strep. pneumoniae* is part of the normal flora of the human respiratory tract but can cause lobar and bronchopneumonia in debilitated patients. *Strep. faecalis* is a normal intestinal inhabitant but may become pathogenic if it gains entry to the blood stream or urinary tract.

Gram-Positive Bacilli

Clostridia

The spore-forming anaerobes consist of many species of clostridia, which are Gram-positive bacilli. The most common human pathogens are *Cl. tetani*, *Cl. perfringens* and *Cl. difficile*.

The natural habitat of *Cl. tetani* is soil, and the usual means of infection is contamination of a wound with soil or manure. Tetanus spores can germinate and release a poison (toxin) under suitable anaerobic conditions. Such conditions are often found in deep lacerations or puncture wounds. However, the causal injury in tetanus may be quite minor.

The effect of the toxin is to increase the excitability of motor neurones so that any movement causes powerful muscle contractions. In severe cases, even a minor movement such as swallowing can provoke a violent contraction, hence the lay term for tetanus, 'lockjaw'.

Although relatively rare now in the UK as a result of immunisation programmes and prophylactic treatment at the time of injury, tetanus remains a serious problem with a high mortality rate in many underdeveloped countries.

Cl. perfringens lives as a commensal in human faeces and is often present on normal skin below the waist. It produces a toxin when carried into wounds involving muscle which has a damaged blood supply. The muscle infection produced is known as **gas gangrene**.

Cl. difficile is sometimes present in normal faeces but its proliferation in the gut is promoted by oral administration of certain antibiotics, notably clindamycin and ampicillin. Proliferation of *Cl. difficile* and production of its toxin may result in the development of a severe infection of the bowel, **pseudomembranous colitis**. The condition is occasionally seen in postoperative patients and requires urgent treatment as it may lead rapidly to death (see chapter 7).

Gram-Negative Cocci

Neisseria

Neisseria are non-motile, non-sporing, Gram-negative, oval diplococci and have a shape somewhat like kidney beans. They are found on mucous membranes, particularly those of the upper respiratory and genitourinary tracts and on the conjunctivae. Most are harmless but *N. gonorrhoea* and *N. meningitidis* are important pathogens.

Neisseria gonorrhoea is transmitted by sexual intercourse and causes urethritis and cervicitis. It can also be transmitted from mother to baby during delivery causing the eye infection ophthalmia neonatorum.

Neisseria meningitidis is often carried in the upper respiratory tract of healthy people but can become pathogenic and cause cerebrospinal meningitis (meningococcal meningitis). Transmission is by direct close contact and epidemics can occur when there is overcrowding, for instance in dormitory conditions. Acute bacterial meningitis can be life-threatening and urgent diagnosis and treatment are necessary. An immediate Gram stain of the cerebrospinal fluid will demonstrate large numbers of Gram-positive diplococci and antibiotic therapy should commence immediately.

Both of these pathogenic organisms die very quickly outside the body and this must be remembered when material for culture is being taken.

Gram-Negative Aerobic Bacilli

Pseudomonas

Pseudomonas aeruginosa can colonise the lower intestinal tract of hospitalised patients, particularly those receiving broad-spectrum antibiotics. It is often considered an opportunistic pathogen, i.e. it can cause infection when the host's defence mechanisms are impaired. It produces a blue–green pus which has a distinctive smell. Most pseudomonas species can be isolated from moist environmental sites in the hospital. The organism often causes severe problems in burns units and intensive therapy units where it can soon contaminate respiratory and other equipment.

Enterobacteria

Enterobacteria are Gram-negative bacilli which may inhabit the intestine of man.

Salmonella   Salmonellae are important intestinal pathogens causing gastroenteritis (see Chapter 10). There are over 700 salmonella species. Poultry is often contaminated with the organism and, if not cooked adequately, can cause outbreaks of infection when eaten. Secondary spread can also occur from person to person if personal hygiene is inadequate.

Shigella   Shigellae cause mild dysentery infections and outbreaks are common in infant nurseries. There are four important shigella species but *Sh. sonnei* and *Sh. flexneri* are the most commonly found in Britain.

Klebsiella   Klebsiella are non-motile, Gram-negative bacilli. *K. aerogenes* is a normal inhabitant of the human intestine but can cause urinary tract, wound and other infections.

Escherichia coli   *E. coli* is a Gram-negative bacillus which is a normal inhabitant of man's intestine. It is the most frequent cause of urinary tract infection and can also present as a pathogen in the respiratory tract of debilitated patients, especially those who have received antibiotic therapy. Some types known as **enteropathogenic**

E. coli can cause gastroenteritis in infants. This can be a fatal condition in debilitated babies.

Proteus and *Serratia* are also Gram-negative bacilli and are fairly common organisms in the hospital environment. Both are able to cause urinary tract and wound infections.

Vibrios

Campylobacter   Poultry is often contaminated by the Gram-negative organism, *C. jejuni*. Transfer to humans results in severe diarrhoea and abdominal pain. According to Shanson (1982), no cases of person-to-person spread have been documented and there is no need to isolate patients with this condition (see chapter 10).

Gram-Negative Anaerobic Bacilli

Bacteroides

Bacteroides is a non-sporing anaerobe commonly found in hospitals. It is a Gram-negative bacillus and dies rapidly in an aerobic environment. This organism is present as part of the normal faecal flora and certain species are found commonly in the female genital tract and mouth.

Bacteroides fragilis is the most common isolate from specimens and can cause abdominal and gynaecological infections.

Acid-Fast Bacteria

Mycobacterium

Mycobacteria are slender bacilli enveloped in a wax coat which makes it difficult to stain them by the Gram method. After staining with hot carbol fuchsin the organisms are stain-fast, resisting decolourisation with alcohols and strong acids. Non-pathogenic forms are widely distributed in nature. *Mycobacterium tuberculosis* and *Mycobacterium bovis* both cause infection in man, the latter being acquired by ingestion of milk from infected cattle.

Tuberculosis is a slow, progressive, chronic infection of the lungs although many other organs and tissues may be affected. The incidence has declined in the Western world but it is still very common in underdeveloped countries. Pulmonary infection is acquired by droplet transmission from a patient with 'open' disease, i.e. one in which tubercle bacilli are found in the sputum. Treatment with antituberculous drugs, such as rifampicin, isoniazid, ethambutol and pyrazinamide, is prolonged but effective.

Mycoplasma

Mycoplasma can be thought of as defective bacteria. They lack a cell wall so have no fixed shape, but are still capable of complete independent metabolic activity. A few species cause disease, such as respiratory illness in man.

Rickettsia and Chlamydia

Rickettsia and chlamydia are prokaryotes that are unable to grow outside a host cell. They are therefore referred to as **obligate intracellular parasites**. Both rickettsia and chlamydia require factors from the host cell to support their growth. Both groups are very difficult to culture in the laboratory.

Rickettsiae are fragile and are not viable when removed from the host cell (the organism that causes Q fever being an exception), and transfer to humans often involves arthropods such as ticks which spread typhus fever.

Chlamydiae are round, slightly smaller than rickettsiae and are responsible for a number of diseases such as pelvic inflammatory disease and non-specific urethritis, both sexually acquired infections.

Viruses

Viruses, like rickettsia and chlamydia, are prokaryotic, obligate intracellular parasites. They are much smaller than other microorganisms and are measured in nanometres (1 nm = 1×10^{-9}m). They range in size from 10–300 nm in diameter. By comparison, a staphylococcus is 1 μm (1000 nm) in diameter. Viruses are too small to be seen with a light microscope and an electron microscope must be used.

In contrast to the other prokaryotes, viruses have very few enzymes and, strictly speaking, no metabolism. They represent the ultimate in specialisation. For their replication they depend on their ability to enter cells of living organisms and to redirect the metabolism of these cells by substituting their own nucleic acid for the cells' DNA. Their dependence on other living cells argues against considering viruses as primitive in the evolutionary sense, that is, as the ancestors of cellular life. Perhaps the simplest notion is that they arose as a sort of parasite at the same time as, or subsequent to, the origin of cellular life. Possibly, some are degenerate forms which have evolved from structures that were once capable of independent life.

Viruses have only one type of nucleic acid, either DNA or RNA. The nuclear material is surrounded by a protein coat or **capsid** that is specific for each type of virus. In some, the capsid and nucleic acid are closely associated and appear to exist in the form of a spiral or **helical** arrangement. In others, the capsid is a shell, clearly separated from the nuclear material, giving the virus a cubic symmetry. This is termed an **icosahedral arrangement** (figure 2.16). The capsid protects the genetic material from destructive enzymes in the environment and also aids attachment of the virus to the host cell. The capsid may be enclosed in an envelope of lipids and

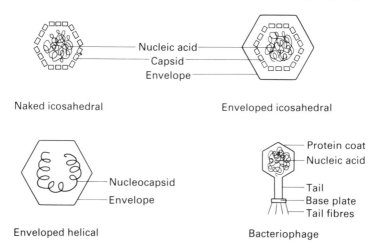

Naked icosahedral   Enveloped icosahedral

Enveloped helical   Bacteriophage

Fig 2.16   Schematic representation of viruses

proteins. Viruses lacking such an envelope are referred to as **naked**.

Infection by virus particles may result in the death of the host cell. Alternatively, the cell may not be killed but may be transformed to become malignant or cancerous. Some viruses produce no obvious effect on the functioning of the cell but remain within it in a latent but potentially infective state, e.g. *herpes zoster*. They may then reactivate and produce a clinical illness; in the case of herpes zoster this is shingles.

Classification of Viruses

There is as yet no entirely satisfactory classification of viruses. In the system described by Timbury (1978), they are assigned to family groups mainly on the basis of the type of nucleic acid and the morphology of the virus particle, and are referred to by the disease they cause. Table 2.4 classifies a number of medically important viruses in this manner.

Viral Replication

Replication of bacteriophages (viruses that infect bacteria) can be used to illustrate the general mechanism of viral replication (figure 2.17, p. 40). Bacteriophages consist of a long thread of DNA packed into a head from which a short tail projects.

1. The virus approaches the bacterial cell and adheres to its surface.

2. The inner core of the tail is thrust through the wall of the bacterium and the DNA strand of the virus is injected into the bacterial cell, similar to the action of a hypodermic syringe.

3. The viral DNA replicates inside the bacterial cell.

Table 2.4 Classification of medically important viruses

Virus Family	Viruses	Disease
DNA Viruses		
Papovaviruses	Papilloma virus	Warts, tumours
Adenoviruses	Adenoviruses	Sore throats, conjunctivitis
Herpes viruses	Herpes simplex I and II	Herpetic skin lesions
	Varicella zoster	Chicken pox and shingles
	Cytomegalovirus	Generalised infections
	Epstein–Barr virus	Glandular fever, Burkitt's lymphoma
Poxviruses	Variola	Smallpox
	Vaccinia	Skin lesions after vaccination
RNA viruses		
Picornaviruses	Enteroviruses	Poliomyelitis, meningitis, respiratory tract infections
	Rhinoviruses	Common colds
Togaviruses	Alphaviruses, Flaviviruses	Anthropod-borne fevers, e.g. yellow fever
Reoviruses	Rotavirus	Gastroenteritis
Rhabdoviruses	Rabies virus	Rabies
Arenaviruses	Lassa fever virus	Lassa fever
	Lymphocytic choriomeningitis	Meningitis
Orthomyxoviruses	Influenza A and B viruses	Influenza
Paramyxoviruses	Para-influenza viruses	Para-influenza
	Respiratory syncytial virus	Bronchiolitis
	Mumps	Mumps
	Measles	Measles
Retroviruses	Human immunodeficiency virus (HIV)	AIDS and related syndromes
	HTLV–1	Leukaemia

4. New virus heads and tails are manufactured and assembled within the cell under the influence of the viral DNA.

5. After about 30 minutes the bacterium bursts open releasing a large number of new virus particles which then repeat the process in other bacterial cells.

The most important of the viral infections seen in hospitals will now be considered in more detail. Although AIDS is caused by a virus it will not be discussed here but is fully covered in chapter 10.

Herpes Simplex Type I

This virus is responsible for the 'cold sore'. Primary infection can occur at any age but it most common in young children, and sores may appear around the mouth and on the conjunctivae and skin. Infections are usually mild and the sores heal completely, but the virus lies dormant in nerve cells and reactivation of the latent virus can occur at times of stress, such as premenstrually or during illness.

Nurses can acquire herpetic whitlows on their fingers from patients with an oral infection, so gloves are recommended for all oral care. Nurses who themselves suffer from herpes infection should not nurse neonates, patients who suffer from chronic eczema or immunosuppressed patients, as these patients are susceptible to generalised herpetic infection which can be fatal.

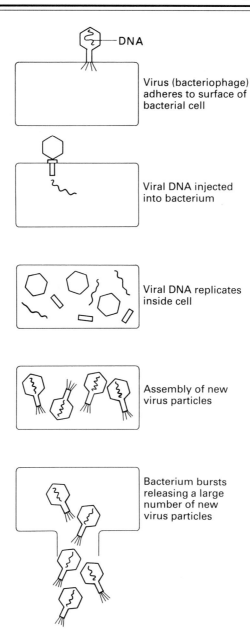

Fig 2.17   Bacteriophage replication

Herpes Zoster

Chickenpox and shingles are both caused by the varicella zoster virus. Following an attack of chickenpox the virus may persist permanently in the sensory nerves and dorsal root ganglia. Reactivation of the latent virus in the form of shingles may occur. Both elderly and immunocompromised patients are prone to develop herpes zoster infections as their natural resistance is lowered. The eruption is infectious and chickenpox can occur in susceptible contacts. Chickenpox is highly infectious and is transmitted by droplet infection. It can be a particular problem on children's wards and among patients whose immune system is compromised.

Viral Hepatitis

Hepatitis A (infectious hepatitis) is transmitted from person to person by faecally contaminated water or food. The disease is endemic in most countries and spreads easily in close contact situations such as in families or schools. Infection may result in abdominal discomfort and fever followed by jaundice. Complete resolution usually occurs.

Hepatitis B (serum hepatitis) is mainly transmitted via the parenteral route, by inoculation of infected blood, although the virus may be present in saliva and semen. Care should be taken when handling body fluids from all patients as asymptomatic infections occur and some people remain 'carriers' following infection. These people are of little risk to other patients but safe disposal of contaminated articles used in their care, for example needles and syringes, should be carried out at all times. Vaccination against hepatitis B is recommended for all staff who are at particular risk of acquiring the illness. The onset of the disease is less apparent than that of hepatitis A and the incubation period is longer. Infection may be asymptomatic, or acute with abdominal pain and jaundice. In a significant proportion of patients, complications such as acute fulminating hepatitis or persistent infection leading to chronic active hepatitis may occur.

Measles

In the UK and other countries where living conditions are of a high standard, the disease is usually mild, but in countries where nutrition levels and living conditions are poor, measles is a serious and frequently fatal disease. In the UK, immunisation is given in childhood to avoid the complications of respiratory tract infections and encephalitis. When a child develops measles after admission to a nursery or hospital ward, it is usual to protect susceptible contacts by administering gamma globulin. This is prepared from pooled human serum (i.e. serum from many donors) obtained from adults who have developed the antibody through childhood exposure to measles.

References

Andrews M L A (1976) *The Life that Lives on Man*. London: Faber and Faber.

Blackwell C and Weir D M (1981) *Principles of Infection and Immunity in Patient Care*. Edinburgh: Churchill Livingstone.

Shanson D C (1982) *Microbiology in Clinical Practice*. Bristol: John Wright.

Timbury M (1978) *Notes on Medical Virology*, 6th edn. Edinburgh: Churchill Livingstone.

Thomas C G A (1979) *Medical Microbiology*, 4th edn. London: Baillière Tindall.

Further Reading

Ayliffe G A J, Collins B J and Taylor L J (1982) *Hospital Acquired Infection: Principles and Prevention*. Bristol: John Wright.

Bell D R (1985) *Lecture Notes on Tropical Medicine*, 2nd edn. Oxford: Blackwell Scientific Publications.

Benenson A S (1985) *Control of Communicable Diseases in Man*. Washington DC: The American Public Health Association.

Mandal B and Mayon-White R T (1984) *Lecture Notes on Infectious Diseases*, 4th edn. Oxford: Blackwell Scientific Publications.

3

The Infection Process

THE TERMINOLOGY OF INFECTION

Microorganisms capable of causing disease are referred to as **pathogens**. Infection results when pathogens have gained access to the tissues, established themselves, multiplied and caused some adverse reaction in the host. Improvements in sanitation, nutrition and housing and the implementation of extensive immunisation programmes have meant that once-feared infectious diseases, such as diphtheria, tuberculosis and smallpox, are now under control. Man generally lives in harmony with the microbial world and only a few of the many species of microorganisms will cause infection in a previously healthy person.

Endogenous (self) infection is caused by microorganisms which originate from the patient himself. Some parts of the body, such as the bladder, are normally free from organisms, i.e. are **sterile**. Other areas, such as the gut, have a natural flora or **commensal** population of microbes. Commensals are harmless in the area where they normally live but, if disturbed, may set up an infection elsewhere in the body. A common example of endogenous infection in the hospitalised patient is urinary tract infection caused by commensal bacteria from the gut. The presence of a catheter increases the likelihood of such an infection as organisms can track along it.

Exogenous infection (or cross-infection) is caused by the transfer to an individual of microorganisms which originate from other people (patients or staff) or from the environment. A hospitalised patient whose natural defence to infection is reduced will be particularly vulnerable to exogenous infection. For example, a patient with an open wound may acquire an exogenous staphylococcal infection by transfer of staphylococcal organisms from a boil or septic lesion of a member of staff.

A pathogen is, as stated above, an organism capable of causing disease. In practice, the definition is somewhat abstract, as an organism may act in a more or less pathogenic manner depending on the circumstances and the response of the host (Shanson, 1982). It is, therefore, helpful if a further classification into conventional, conditional and opportunistic pathogens is made.

Conventional pathogens are capable of causing infection in a previously healthy person. Such microorganisms are not usually part of the normal or commensal flora and spread usually occurs from infected cases or carriers. An example of a conventional pathogen is *Streptococcus pyogenes* which can cause a number of infections ranging from sore throats to scarlet fever.

Conditional pathogens are capable of causing infection under some circumstances. Often, such microorganisms are part of the commensal flora but, if disturbed from their normal site, they can set up an infection elsewhere. For example, bacteroides is a commensal organism of the gut but can act as a conditional pathogen if disturbed and may be responsible for wound infections following abdominal surgery.

Some organisms will only cause an infection when the body's defence system is impaired. These are appropriately referred to as **opportunistic** pathogens. An example of such an organism is *Pneumocystitis carinii* which causes the respiratory infection ofen seen in patients with acquired immune deficiency syndrome (AIDS). This severe respiratory tract infection only develops if a patient's immune response is impaired, as it is in AIDS.

When the response to invasion by pathogens is slight, or even absent, there is said to be **colonisation** rather than infection. For example, a laboratory report from a leg ulcer swab may record a growth of *Staphylococcus aureus*. If the ulcer is infected, the growth of *Staph. aureus* will be associated with a tissue reaction such as inflammation and the production of pus. However, if on examination the ulcer appears healthy, colonisation and not infection has occurred. A laboratory report is useful, but it is the careful observation and reporting by the nurse dressing the ulcer that will determinate whether any specific treatment is necessary. This is not to say that colonisation, particularly in the hospitalised patient, is unimportant. Colonisation may indicate that an organism is spreading in a ward or unit and, in the case of very resistant organisms like methicillin-resistant *Staph. aureus* (MRSA), the situation is potentially dangerous as the organism can spread from colonised patients to cause infection in others. MRSA has been responsible for large outbreaks of hospital-acquired infection necessitating the closure of wards or units to bring the problem under control (see chapter 10).

ROUTES OF MICROBIAL TRANSMISSION

The process by which infection can be spread from one susceptible host to another can be thought of as a continuous chain. All links must be maintained, and in the proper order, for the chain to remain intact and infection to be transmitted to another individual (figure 3.1).

The Causative Organism

To break the chain of infection, the causative organism must be destroyed or rendered harmless. In the hospital setting, many infection control measures, e.g. disinfection or sterilisation of equipment, are aimed at removing this link. For example, nurses can prevent cross-infection by practising good research-based nursing such as using individual, dry wash-bowls for patients (Greaves, 1985). Sometimes, breaking this link in the chain is less easy as in the case of an outbreak of influenza in the community.

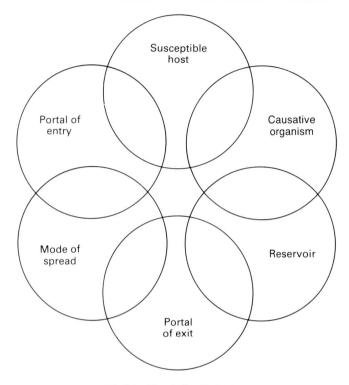

Fig 3.1   The chain of infection

The Reservoir

In a hospital, dust, insects and vermin may all act as reservoirs and a clean hospital environment will remove this link. A patient or member of hospital staff may also act as a reservoir of infection. Any infection in staff should be reported immediately and all new patients observed for signs of infection, such as boils, infected eczema, infected wounds or fever.

The Portals of Entry and Exit

The route by which a pathogen leaves its host is called the portal of exit, and the route by which it enters is called the portal of entry. The main portals of entry are:

- *The respiratory tract*, through inhalation of organisms (e.g. in tuberculosis, diphtheria and mumps)
- *The alimentary tract*, through ingestion of contaminated food or water (e.g. in dysentery, poliomyelitis and salmonellosis)
- *The skin and mucous membranes*, either by the passage of organisms through damaged skin as with infected wounds, or by the inoculation of organisms (e.g. in hepatitis B transferred from contaminated needles)

● *The placenta*, via transfer of organisms from the maternal to the foetal circulation (e.g. for rubella, cytomegalovirus and syphilis)

There are a number of routes by which infectious agents can leave the host. The exit route may be the same as that of entry, e.g. the respiratory tract in tuberculosis, or a different route, as in salmonella infections where the route of entry is usually via the mouth and the exit route is in the faeces.

Mode of Spread

Infection can be transferred in the following ways.

● Direct personal contact with contaminated body secretions or excretions, particularly via staff hands that have become contaminated
● Indirect contact with contaminated equipment such as shaving brushes, needles and syringes
● Vectors such as cockroaches, fleas, flies, mosquitoes and other insects that harbour infectious agents
● Airborne spread of contaminated skin scales and spread through an aerosol of contaminated droplets from patients' sneezing and coughing
● Endogenous spread from one part of a person's body to another part

Of these, direct personal contact, particularly hand contamination, is the most important. Modes of spread may be interconnected, hand contact often providing this link (figure 3.2). This is why hand-washing is stressed as the most important measure in reducing cross-infection (see chapters 5 and 8). Appendix II lists some of the more important infections with their associated chains of infection, and nursing intervention to break the chain of infection will be discussed in chapter 8.

Susceptible Host

For infection to occur once an organism has reached its target, the host must be susceptible. The competence of the body's innate and acquired defence mechanisms will affect whether or not illness occurs and the chain of infection may also be broken at this point.

HOST DEFENCE MECHANISMS

The concept and study of immunity go back a long way in history. The Romans were aware that those who had recovered from an outbreak of plague could safely nurse new cases. Nowadays, we are aware that an attack of measles encountered in childhood will give life-long protection against a further attack, but it will not provide any protection against an unrelated infection such as chickenpox. We are also aware that the body has certain natural barriers against infection, such as the

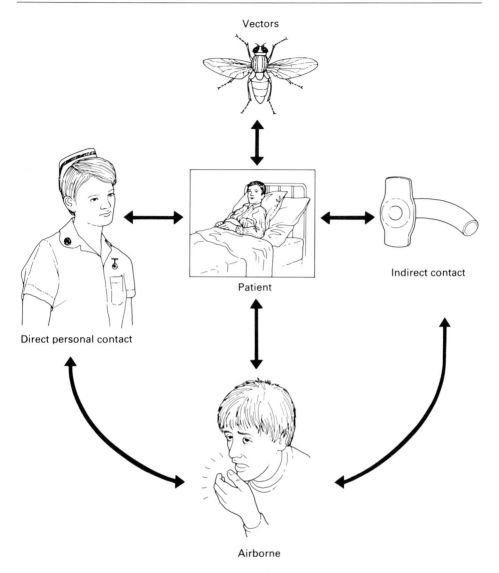

Fig 3.2 The role of hands in the spread of infection

skin. If the skin is cut or damaged infection can ensue. **Non-specific defence mechanisms** are natural barriers which protect against invasion by pathogens. **Specific immune mechanisms** are activated if an organism, for instance the measles virus, is able to evade the non-specific defence system. This specific response may not prevent an attack but will ensure that a memory of the measles virus is retained so that the system can react quickly and destroy the virus when it is next encountered.

Non-Specific Defence Mechanisms

These are dependent on the following:

- The skin and normal body flora
- Mucous membranes, secretion and mechanical washings
- Genetic make-up
- Nutritional status and hormonal influences
- Inflammation and phagocytosis

The Skin and Normal Body Flora

An intact skin is the most important defence against microbial invasion. Any break such as a cut or burn will expose the host to a risk of infection, as will malnutrition or extreme dampness of the skin.

Apart from acting as a mechanical barrier the skin has a low pH, and this acid environment is inhibitory to many pathogenic bacteria. The natural microbial flora of the skin help to prevent colonisation or invasion by more pathogenic organisms. The consequences of disturbances in this equilibrium are evident in the hospitalised patient. When broad spectrum antibiotics are used they can wipe out the normal flora which are then replaced by potentially more harmful organisms. In hospitals, candida (thrush) infection of the mouth is common when antibiotics have inhibited the normal oral flora (Ayliffe et al, 1982).

A number of body systems are defended by the presence of normal flora. Table 3.1 gives examples of the normal (commensal) body flora in important organs and tissues.

Mucous Membranes, Secretions and Mechanical Washings

Mucous membranes provide an obvious route of entry for microorganisms into the host. Often this is achieved by the organism attaching to the epithelial cells of the mucosa; *Neisseria gonorrhoea*, for example, attaches to the epithelial cells of the genitourinary tract by the pili on its surface. In order to prevent invasion, mucosal surfaces need to repel attachment and remove invading organisms from the body. This applies particularly to those membranes exposed to the outside environment: the eyes, respiratory tract, vagina, gastrointestinal tract and urinary tract.

Various mechanical structures, such as mucus-covered cilia in the respiratory tract, help in this process. In this example, attachment to the epithelium is prevented when organisms are trapped in mucus and swept out by the constant movement of the cilia. If this step is evaded, coughing or sneezing can remove organisms attached to the mucosa.

Additional help is provided by antibacterial substances such as lysozyme and antibodies present in mucosal secretions. Secretions may be acid (e.g. gastric juice), contain fatty acids (e.g. sweat) or be strongly alkaline (e.g. bile). These substances help to selectively promote the normal flora at the expense of pathogens.

Table 3.1   Normal body flora

Site	Organism
Skin	Staphylococcus epidermidis Micrococci Diphtheroids
Upper respiratory tract	Streptococcus viridans Diphtheroids Neisseriae catarrhalis
Stomach	Normally sterile
Intestine	Bacteroides spp. Escherichia coli Streptococcus faecalis Proteus spp. Clostridia Lactobacilli Yeasts
Kidney and bladder	Normally sterile
Female genital tract	Lactobacilli Coliforms Staphylococcus epidermidis

Genetic Make-Up

Differences in susceptibility to infectious agents due to genetic factors are well known (Blackwell and Weir, 1981). Diseases may be species-specific such as distemper which is seen in dogs but not in man. Differences are also seen among members of a single species, as with the increased susceptibility of some human races to tuberculosis. It has even been shown that if one homozygous twin develops tuberculosis, the other twin has a 3 to 1 chance of developing the disease compared with a 1 in 3 chance for a heterozygous twin.

Nutritional Status and Hormonal Influences

Poor nutrition affects every component of the defence system. In addition, poor diet is often associated with poor environmental conditions which may lead to increased exposure to infection.

Patients with diseases such as diabetes mellitus and hypothyroidism, and those requiring steroid therapy, have also been shown to be at increased risk of infection. The reasons for this are not entirely clear, although the anti-inflammatory properties of steroids are known to decrease the ability of phagocytes (cells that destroy invading organisms) to act.

There is increasing research emerging that emotional states, particularly stress, can greatly affect disease susceptibility and immune responsiveness. Most studies have been carried out among cancer patients but results of further research could have important implications for nursing practice, particularly for the physiological care of the patient (Boore, 1978). As an exercise five patients can be chosen from the ward and the possible factors that would put them at increased risk of infection listed.

Inflammation and Phagocytosis

Once a microorganism has gained access to the tissues, it will proliferate at the site of infection, and this will result in a local inflammatory response. The signs of inflammation are heat, redness, swelling and tenderness or pain, and these signs will be similar whether the tissue irritant is an organism, a foreign body or a chemical. Changes are induced in the permeability of the blood vessels at the site of infection. This results in an out-pouring of serum, phagocytic cells and some red cells from the blood vessels into the tissues. Phagocytic cells are able to take up particulate materials by a process known as phagocytosis and soluble substances by a progress known as **pinocytosis**. The cells of the blood and immune system are illustrated in figure 3.3.

There are two types of phagocytic cells: **mononuclear** (with a single nucleus) and **polymorphonuclear** (multinucleate). The mononuclear phagocytes include both circulating blood **monocytes** and **macrophages** found in various tissues of the body. The mononuclear phagocytes arise from bone marrow **stem cells** and, after proliferation and maturation, pass into the blood as monocytes. After about 24 hours they migrate to their main site of action in the tissues where they differentiate into macrophages. Here they can divide and are capable of surviving for many months. Polymorphonuclear phagocytes (**neutrophils**) also arise from bone marrow stem cells and, after about 12 hours in the blood, enter the tissue where they quickly die. The release of phagocytic cells and serum into the tissues in the inflammatory response brings them into contact with the invading organisms.

Some substances in serum such as the **interferons** and **transferrin** are able to kill or suppress the growth of organisms. Interferons are a family of proteins that are important in non-specific defence mechanisms against viral infection. They are released from virally infected cells and taken up by other cells, providing protection from the invading virus and, often, other related viral infections. Transferrin is an iron-binding protein in the serum. Bacteria are dependent on iron, so compete with transferrin to obtain it; their growth will be inhibited in serum containing high levels of transferrin and low levels of iron.

Certain other substances in serum are able to attach non-specifically to the surface of many organisms. After further interactions with yet another series of serum factors, the **complement system**, this can lead to the important event of **phagocytosis** in which the bacterium is ingested and destroyed (figure 3.4).

The complement system is a complex enzymatic system composed of a series of proteins which interact in a sequence or 'cascade' fashion, rather like a line of dominoes knocking each other over (Kirkwood and Lewis, 1983). Organisms may become coated with derivatives of one of the complement components known as C_3; such a factor attaching to a bacterium to increase phagocytosis is called an **opsonin**. The organisms then adhere strongly to the membranes of phagocytic cells which have a binding site or **receptor** for C_3. This attachment of such opsonised

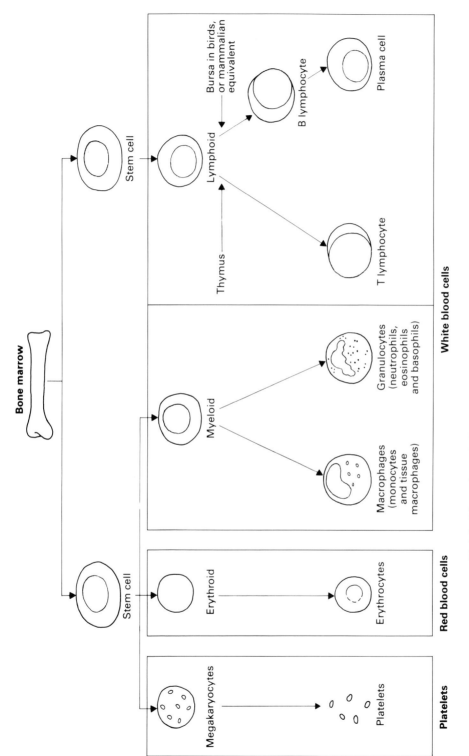

Fig 3.3 Maturation and differentiation of cells of the blood and immune system

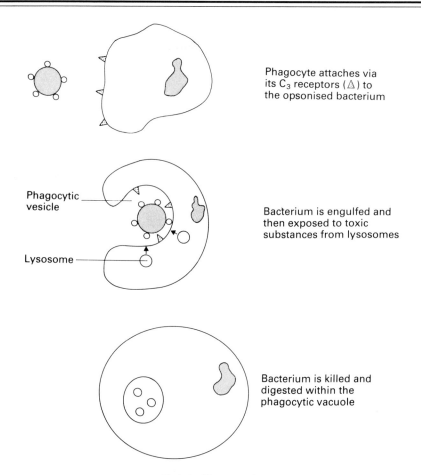

Phagocyte attaches via
its C_3 receptors ($\triangle$) to
the opsonised bacterium

Phagocytic
vesicle

Lysosome

Bacterium is engulfed and
then exposed to toxic
substances from lysosomes

Bacterium is killed and
digested within the
phagocytic vacuole

Fig 3.4   Phagocytosis

organisms to phagocytes greatly increases the efficiency with which they can be engulfed. Indeed, C_3 is so important that congenital absence of it leads to rapid death from infection. C_3 also promotes the enzymatic modification of other components of the complement system, which then become active as chemotoxins and attract more phagocytic cells to the site of infection. Another group of complement components is able to lyse cell membranes, and a few species of bacteria and viruses can be killed directly by this lytic pathway.

   Engulfment by phagocytes results in organisms being exposed to toxic molecules and destructive enzymes which usually kill them although, occasionally, the pathogens are able to kill the phagocytes. This process may be identified by the production of **pus** – an accumulation of living and dead phagocytes, cell debris and organisms.

   If microorganisms survive these non-specific defence mechanisms, proliferation may lead to local abscess formation or spread via the lymphatics to other parts of the body. Some organisms like *Corynebacterium diphtheriae* produce **exotoxins** (external toxins) which will have damaging effects throughout the body without the spread of bacteria from the initial site of infection. Other bacteria, such as tubercle bacilli, damage local tissue by entering and infecting it. Toxigenic organisms tend to produce acute, short-lived infective states, while intracellular organisms cause chronic infective states.

Specific Defence Mechanisms

As previously described, non-specific defence mechanisms deal with potentially harmful materials on the host's first and subsequent exposures to them. Although specific immune responses are activated during the host's first exposure, it is only on subsequent exposures that the system can provide an effective defence mechanism. Taking the example of measles, the host's non-specific defence mechanisms are generally not effective in preventing infection. A specific immune response is activated on the first exposure and is brought into play on subsequent exposures. This system offers a high degree of protection and second attacks of measles are rare.

Tissues and Cells of the Immune System

The tissues of the immune system comprise the spleen, lymph nodes and gut-associated lymphoid tissue (Peyer's patches and appendix, figure 3.5). Foreign material is conveyed to the spleen via the bloodstream and to the lymph nodes via the lymphatics, the small lymph containing vessels which drain the tissues.

Two types of cells, **phagocytes** and **lymphocytes**, take part in the specific immune response. These cells originate in the bone marrow. Some lymphocytes migrate from the bone marrow into the thymus gland and mature there before passing to the lymphoid tissue of gut, spleen and lymph nodes or into the blood where they are known as **T lymphocytes (T cells)**. Bone marrow-derived lymphocytes that differentiate in the bursal equivalent tissue are known as **B lymphocytes (B cells)**. The bursal equivalent tissue is so called because the site of maturation, originally discovered in birds to be the bursal sac, has not yet been located in man.

B lymphocytes can recognise certain substances as being foreign and, when this happens, the cells become metabolically active. They divide and eventually give rise to **plasma cells**. Plasma cells in turn produce families of proteins known as **antibodies** or **immunoglobulins**. T lymphocytes cannot differentiate into plasma cells. Their importance is in recognising foreign material that is inside cells or fixed in tissue.

In summary **B** lymphocytes are responsible for the antibody mediated or **humoral** immune response. They differentiate in the bursal equivalent tissue and protect the host from bacterial infection.

T lymphocytes are responsible for **cell-mediated** immunity. They develop in the thymus and protect the host from tumours, tuberculosis and other intracellular infections (particularly viral), and are important in transplant rejection.

Although they are closely related, humoral and cell-mediated immunity will be discussed separately.

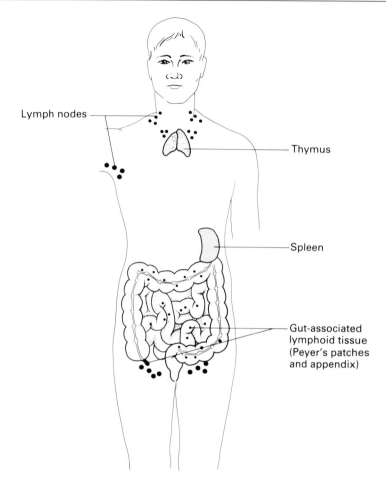

Fig 3.5   Organs and tissues of the immune system

Humoral Immunity

The humoral immune response is activated following stimulation of the immune system by an **antigen**. An antigen is defined as any substance which is capable of stimulating the formation of antibody and the development of cell-mediated immunity. The stimulating substance must appear to be foreign to the body. The body can usually distinguish between self and non-self correctly, although occasionally this natural tolerance is disturbed, as seen in autoimmune disease.

Antibodies are able to neutralise antigens by combining with them. The binding of the antigen to the antibody binding site is like a 'lock and key' mechanism (figure 3.6). Antibodies of different degrees of specificity (exactness) may be produced in the immune response to a given antigen. Only a well-fitting 'lock' will neutralise a given antigen. Some antigens can combine as a 'poor fit' with antibody produced to a completely different antigen, which can have clinical implications. For example, in acute rheumatic fever antibody produced against a *Streptococcus pyogenes*

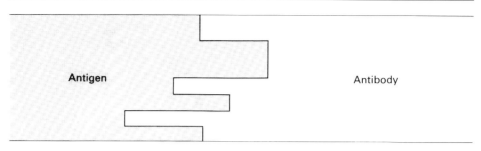

Good fit of 'lock' leads to neutralisation of antigen

Fig 3.6   Antigen–antibody binding: the 'lock and key' mechanism

infection in the throat may cross-react with heart tissue (which is incorrectly recognised by the antibody as antigen) leading to myocarditis and valvular disease.

Antibodies are divided into five main classes each of which has different properties; they are referred to collectively as **immunoglobulins**. The roles of the classes IgG, IgA, IgM, IgD, IgE are summarised in table 3.2.

Table 3.2   Immunoglobulins

IgG	Main immunoglobulin of the secondary immune response. Small molecule of high specificity. Will readily diffuse into interstitial fluid and across the placenta. Important in the neutralisation of toxins and precipitation of antigens
IgA	Main immunoglobulin of the external secretory system. Present in saliva, tears, breast milk, respiratory and intestinal fluid. Important role in protection of mucosal surfaces
IgM	Main immunoglobulin of the primary immune response. Large molecule of five units with a low specificity. Important in agglutination and complement fixation
IgE	IgE-producing cells found in respiratory intestinal mucosa. Important role as the mediator of allergic reactions
IgD	Membrane-associated immunoglobulin. Role unclear

The basic antibody molecule consists of two identical heavy chains and two light chains, held together by a chemical link (figure 3.7). The five antibody classes are distinguished by their heavy chains. The Fab portion of the antibody contains the variable regions of the molecule and provides the 'lock', i.e. it allows the antibody to attach specifically to a particular type of antigen. The constant Fc portion differs from one class of antibody to another, and the structure of the heavy chain constant portion serves as a basis for distinguishing the classes of antibody.

Antibody Response

Exposure to antigen is followed by a latent period when there is no detectable antibody in the blood. On first exposure, a latent period of two to four days is followed by a primary response with rapid rise of antibodies, initially IgM and then IgG, the latter being more specific and so providing a better 'lock'. On secondary

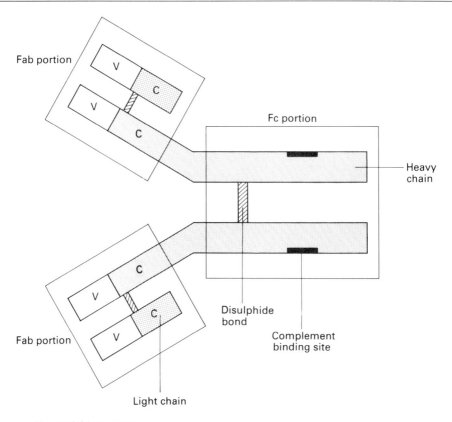

Fig 3.7   Structure of the basic antibody molecule

exposure, fast production and high levels of specific IgG antibody are achieved due to activation of the memory of the previous exposure.

Antigen is first processed by receptors on T lymphocytes which stimulate B cells which in turn produce antibodies. Some lymphocytes remain as memory cells. Antibody helps to protect the host in the following ways:

1. Secretion of antibody into the bronchi, gut and tears reinforces the non-specific barriers such as mucus and cilia. Secretion into maternal milk helps to provide protection for babies while they develop their own immune responses.

2. Antibody can neutralise the effects of toxins by combining with the active part of the toxin.

3. Antibody can cover a virus thereby blocking its ability to attach to the surface of a cell. This will prevent entry into the cell and hence infection.

4. Antibody molecules have at least two combining sites (see figure 3.7), so can combine with more than one antigen. The resulting agglutination of, for instance, viruses will enhance their engulfment by phagocytic cells.

5. The complement system can be activated by the attachment of antibody molecules to antigen on an organism's surface (see above). Some organisms will be lysed directly by the attachment of these complement components.

6. Phagocytic cells have receptors on their membranes for the free Fc end of the antibody molecule. There are also receptors for the complement component, C_3, which often coats organisms. Both mechanisms enhance adhesion of the antigen to the cell and thus promote phagocytosis.

Cell-Mediated Immune Response

A cell-mediated immune response is required to protect the host from viral infections, some fungal infections and parasitic diseases, and intracellular bacteria. In these situations the antigen is inaccessible as it is inside the host cell and antigen–antibody reactions appear to be relatively inefficient. Cell-mediated immunity is also responsible for delayed hypersensitivity, transplant rejection and tumour surveillance.

The response is dependent on T lymphocytes rather than on the B lymphocytes of the humoral immune response, and is initiated by the binding of antigen with an antigen receptor on the surface of a sensitised T lymphocyte. If a T cell encounters an antigen which its receptors recognise, it may release mediators known as **lymphokines.** The lymphokines activate macrophages in the vicinity, resulting in an enhancement of phagocytosis.

T cells proliferate and can differentiate into a variety of effector T cells. Some of these are **cytotoxic T lymphocytes** which specifically destroy any target cell with an appropriate surface antigen, such as virus-infected cells which may express viral antigens on their surface, or cancerous cells which may have altered antigenically. Still others control the responses of various other antigen-triggered lymphocytes, either as **helpers** that promote the maturation of antigen-stimulated B and T cells, or as **suppressors** that block the enhancing activity of the T helpers (figure 3.8).

Another cell type, not a T cell or B cell, can also play a part in cell-mediated immunity. This is the **killer** or K cell, whose precise origin and role are unknown. It can recognise and destroy antibody coated target cells. Whereas a T lymphocyte needs to be sensitised before it can react to a 'foreign' cell, a K cell does not.

Control of the Immune Response

The complex reaction of the immune response is controlled both genetically and by a cellular interaction. Genetic influences can be observed between different species in the production of antibody to a given antigen. Within species, some genetic types have been found to be good antibody producers while others react poorly.

Control at the cellular level is largely by the T cells, notably helper and suppressor T cells, which play an important role in cellular control in both humoral and cell-mediated immunity. Helper T cells can interact with an antigen to release substances which help B lymphocytes to produce antibodies against this antigen. Suppressor T cells stem this response. In the normal immune response a fine

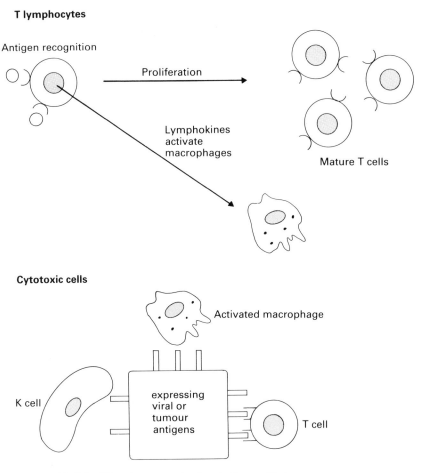

Fig 3.8   T lymphocyte mechanisms in the specific immune response

balance is reached between the action of helper and suppressor T cells, and any imbalance can have serious consequences.

THE COMPROMISED HOST

Genetic abnormalities of the primary immune system are seen in some children who suffer from repeated infections of chest, ear and, in some cases, joints. However, defects may be acquired at any stage in life as a result of bacterial or viral infections. For example, the herpes simplex virus can infect macrophages, ensuring the continuation of the virus and a reduced response by the host to other infections. Spreading tumour cells can replace lymphoid tissue, and immunosuppressive drugs or radiation therapy will render a patient highly susceptible to infection. Diabetes or steroid therapy will also result in immunosuppression.

Some patients, although not compromised by outside influences, may also be at an increased risk of infection. These patients include the very old and the very young in whom the immune system is not fully active. In fact, any breach in the normal host defence mechanism will render a person more open to infection. This was illustrated in a large research study of surgical wound infections conducted by Cruse and Ford (1980). They quantified the risk of acquiring a wound infection as:

$$\text{Risk of infection} = \frac{\text{Dose of bacterial contamination} \times \text{Virulence}}{\text{Resistance of the host}}$$

They demonstrated that any factors which lowered the resistance of the host would alter the equation, so that infection could occur even if the dose of bacterial contamination was lowered or the pathogen was less virulent. When a very virulent pathogen is encountered, e.g. the first exposure to measles virus, infection can result even when the resistance of the host is quite high.

VACCINATION AND IMMUNISATION

Specific or **acquired** immunity can be brought about in a number of ways (figure 3.9). **Active** exposure to an infectious agent can result in a clinical infection or an asymptomatic (sub-clinical) infection, both of which can confer immunity. **Passive** transfer of immunity from an immunised individual to an unimmunised person can occur through blood serum transfer of antibodies or lymphocytes.

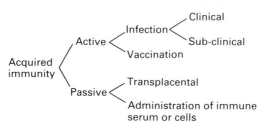

Fig 3.9 The acquired immune response

Immunity can also be actively initiated by vaccination. Vaccines and antitoxins are produced from the following:

● Killed organisms, e.g. the vaccine against typhoid
● Attenuated (modified) organisms, e.g. for BCG vaccination against tuberculosis
● Modified exotoxins, e.g. against diphtheria

Vaccines can give protection against a wide variety of infections (figure 3.10). Detailed information on recommendations and requirements for immunisation is published by the Department of Health. Recommendations for those travelling abroad vary each year and guidelines are given in appropriate leaflets which can be obtained from local Department of Health offices.

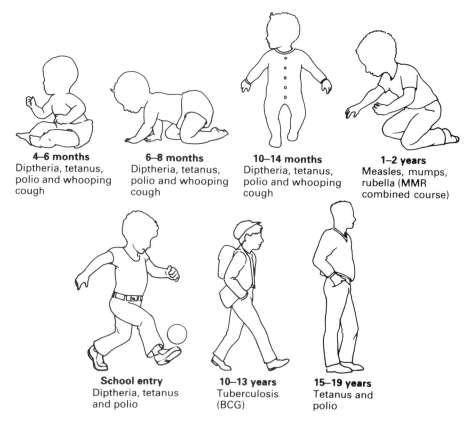

4–6 months
Diptheria, tetanus,
polio and whooping
cough

6–8 months
Diptheria, tetanus,
polio and whooping
cough

10–14 months
Diptheria, tetanus,
polio and whooping
cough

1–2 years
Measles, mumps,
rubella (**MMR**
combined course)

School entry
Diptheria, tetanus
and polio

10–13 years
Tuberculosis
(BCG)

15–19 years
Tetanus and
polio

Fig 3.10   The recommended UK immunisation schedule

References

Ayliffe G A J, Collins B J and Taylor L J (1982) *Hospital Acquired Infection: Principles and Prevention*. Bristol: John Wright.

Blackwell C and Weir D M (1981) *Principles of Infection and Immunity in Patient Care*. Edinburgh: Churchill Livingstone.

Boore J (1978) *A Prescription for Recovery*. RCN Research Series. London: Royal College of Nursing.

Cruse J E and Ford R (1980) The epidemiology of wound infection. *Surgical Clinics of North America*, **60**: 27–39.

Greaves A (1985) 'We'll just freshen you up, dear . . .'. *Nursing Times*, **81**(10), *Journal of Infection Control Nursing*, pp. 3–8.

Kirkwood E and Lewis C (1983) *Understanding Medical Immunology*. Chichester: John Wiley and Sons.

Shanson D C (1982) *Microbiology in Clinical Practice*. Bristol: John Wright.

Further Reading

Bannister B (1983) *Infectious Diseases*. London: Baillière Tindall.
Parker M J and Stucke V A (1982) *Microbiology for Nurses*. London: Baillière Tindall.
Weir D M (1983) *Immunology: An Outline for Students of Medicine and Biology*, 5th edn. Edinburgh: Churchill Livingstone.

Hospital- and
Community Acquired Infection

Hospitals are a vital part of the UK health-care system and arise from the need to centralise clinical facilities, manpower and money. The effective organisation and management of these assembled resources should provide the public with an efficient hospital service. In material and financial terms the advantages of hospital-orientated health care may be obvious, but what of the disadvantages?

HOSPITAL-ACQUIRED INFECTION

By the very nature of its work, a hospital constantly exposes patients to microbiological risks. When a person enters hospital, he exchanges his secure home environment for a bed in a small, possibly restricted, hostile area – the ward. From the moment of admission to hospital the person is potentially put at a disadvantage by his illness, environment, medication, surgery and other treatment.

The attendant risk of spread of infection from others is compounded by sharing facilities, equipment and staff with other patients of similar diagnosis undergoing common intervention and treatment. It may seem strange that, in an effort to cure, we take people from the safety of their homes and expect them to make progress in the comparatively unsafe environment of a hospital. Fortunately, the current trend towards day surgery, day centres, community orientated care and shorter stays in hospital should lessen the length of, or in the same instances remove the need for, hospitalisation, and thus cut down the risk of a patient contracting a hospital acquired infection (HAI).

Definition of HAI

Hospital-acquired infection (HAI) is defined as infection which is acquired by patients while they are in hospital or by staff who are working in the hospital. It is often referred to as nosocomial infection, from the Greek words 'nosos' (disease) and 'komeo' (attend to). If patients acquire infection more than 72 hours after admission, it is considered to be hospital-acquired rather than community acquired infection.

Incidence and Prevalence of HAI

The incidence rate of a condition is established by the continuous recording of the number of cases over a defined period of time. Approximately 10 per cent of people admitted to hospital in the UK contract an HAI; thus the incidence rate is 10 per cent. Prevalence rates are not obtained from continuous recording but, instead, register the number of HAIs present at the time of the survey. At any one time, about 20 per cent of patients in hospital are suffering from HAI, i.e. the prevalence rate is 20 per cent. Prevalence rates are about double incidence rates because the patient with an HAI extends his hospital stay.

In 1980, the first national prevalence study of infection was undertaken in England and Wales (Meers et al, 1981). This large prevalence study involved 18 163 patients in 43 hospitals (table 4.1). The study showed that 19.1 per cent of patients were infected. Over half of these (51.9 per cent) were community acquired infections (CAIs) and the rest (48.1 per cent) were HAIs.

As stated above, 10 per cent of patients admitted to hospital in the UK with no evidence of infection contract an infection as a result of their admission. In America, the nationwide nosocomial infection rate is given as approximately 5.7 infections per 100 admissions (Haley et al, 1985).

In addition to this, hospital-acquired infection can be either endemic or epidemic. **Endemic** refers to the continuous and constant incidence of infection caused by local factors, e.g. the type of patient, the length of his stay in hospital and the type of surgery he is undergoing. An **epidemic** infection is one caused by a substantial increase in the rate of endemic infections or by the appearance of an organism not normally present to the presence of an infected person or carrier or,

Table 4.1 Survey of the prevalence of infection

	Community acquired infections %	Hospital-acquired infections %	All infections %
Lower respiratory	31.6	16.8	24.5
Upper respiratory	6.3	3.2	4.8
Urinary	14.5	30.3	22.1
Skin	18.6	13.5	16.2
Minor wound	0.8	11.0	5.7
Major wound	0.8	7.9	4.2
Female genital	4.0	4.0	4.0
Bones and joints	3.2	2.5	2.9
Eye	2.2	3.5	2.8
Gastrointestinal	2.6	1.4	2.0
Bacteraemia	1.6	1.1	1.4
Gangrenous foot	1.5	0.7	1.1
CNS	1.7	0.3	1.0
Ear	1.3	0.4	0.9
Other	9.2	3.5	6.5
Total number of infections	1802	1671	3473

(From Meers et al, 1981. Reproduced by kind permission of the *Journal of Hospital Infection.*)

fortunately rarely these days, to contaminated fluids such as cleansing lotions and multiple-dose drugs. One reported epidemic infection (Ayliffe et al, 1983) resulted in 15 infections among 25 patients, all of whom had been subjected to intraocular operations in the same week. Six of these patients lost the sight of one eye.

Microbiology of HAI

The organisms responsible for hospital-acquired infection are constantly changing. In the 1930s, infection caused by haemolytic streptococci was the main problem. Following the introduction of sulphonamide and penicillin antibiotics, *Staph. aureus* became the major hazard. In the early 1960s, these Gram-positive organisms assumed less importance as Gram-negative organisms became prevalent in hospitals. Since the beginning of the 1980s, Gram-positive organisms, especially antibiotic-resistant *Staph. aureus*, have again been increasing in incidence (Meers et al, 1981). Figure 4.1 outlines the organisms now commonly causing HAI.

THE RISK OF ACQUIRING AN HAI

In order to assess how much impact hospital microorganisms might have on a

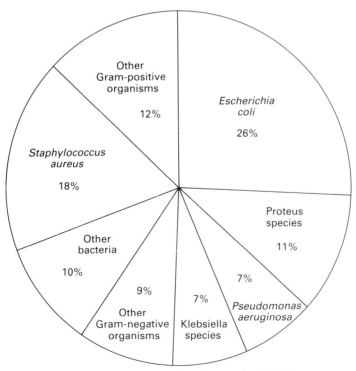

Fig 4.1   Common causes of hospital-acquired infection

person, we need to look at:

● General factors associated with the hospital itself
● Personal factors associated with the response that the individual is able to mount

The outcome of exposure to infection is related to both sets of factors (table 4.2).

Hospital-Related Factors

Contact with an Infected Person

A hospital is, by definition, a place to which the sick are brought for treatment. A patient with a contagious disease or other type of infection becomes a potential source of cross-infection when he is admitted to hospital. Any in-patient could be exposed to the causative microorganism, but, for the already vulnerable patient, this exposure adds a further element of risk.

Contact with Other People

The hospital is a hive of activity. The sheer number of people contained within this limited area, and their close and constant exchanges, favours the spread of microorganisms. All staff and patients carry their own microbial flora and some of these people will, additionally, be healthy carriers of pathogenic bacteria.

Hospital-based contact tracing exercises tend to demonstrate that the estimated number of personal interactions falls far short of the actual number of contacts. One such example (unpublished) concerns two ladies on a ward caring for elderly people who were found to be excretors of *Salmonella indiana*. The probability of person-to-person spread having been established, stool specimens were requested from the other patients and all staff who had been in close contact with the two ladies during the previous seven days. This request produced 166 contacts: 4 doctors, 1 housekeeper, 4 physiotherapists, 1 voluntary worker, 1 hairdresser, 4 occupational therapists, 25 domestic workers, 83 nurses, 34 patients and 9 bedmakers. This, however, was not the actual total as visitors and 'casual' contacts were excluded from the screening exercise.

Table 4.2 Factors influencing the risk of infection
from exposure to hospital microorganisms

Hospital-related factors	
● Contact with an infected person	● Antibiotic-resistant microorganisms
● Contact with many other people	● Bypassing of natural defences

Personal factors	
● Immunity status	● Psychosocial well-being
● Age	● Underlying disease
● Physical well-being	● Medical intervention

Antibiotic-Resistant Microorganisms

Antibiotic administration to both patients and staff can lead to the suppression of relatively antibiotic-sensitive organisms in favour of highly resistant strains. In this way, antibiotics can 'select out' and encourage the multiplication of resistant microbial strains which can then colonise an individual or an area of the hospital. This results in the creation of an animal or environmental reservoir.

For example, methicillin-resistant *Staphylococcus aureus* (MRSA) cross-infection may occur between patients in an intensive care unit (ICU). A screening programme will be set up, and it may be that MRSA will be detected in the environment. This, of course, has implications for the standard of cleanliness, but the frequent prescribing of broad-spectrum antibiotics for ICU patients will be a contributory factor in the establishment of the environmental MRSA reservoir.

Antibiotic-resistant bacteria tend to become endemically established in line with local antibiotic prescribing patterns. The removal of antibiotic-sensitive flora may result in a smaller than normal inoculum of organisms being able to cause infection. Prolonged colonisation can also be demonstrated by the prolonged excretion of enteric pathogens such as salmonella.

Bypassing of Natural Defences

Any procedure which bypasses the natural defences of the body heightens the possibility of infection. As long as it remains intact, the skin is the body's most effective barrier to microorganisms.

All invasive procedures carry with them the risk of introducing microorganisms into the body, and no procedure breaches the skin's integrity more extensively than does surgery. The introduction of such devices as central venous cannulae, intravenous needles and urinary catheters creates potential pathways for bacteria to enter the body. Specialised care units increase the risk of disease as the equipment used frequently bypasses normal defences. ICUs are good examples of this, as a proportion of their patients will be artificially ventilated and parenterally fed, as well as having continuous bladder drainage.

Personal Factors Associated with Resistance

Immunity Status

Immunity may be natural or acquired and will vary between individuals. (See chapter 3 for a fuller discussion.)

Age

In old age, with natural impairment of function, the immune system becomes less efficient. At the other end of the scale, an infant's immune mechanism will not be fully developed.

Physical Well-Being

A person who is in a state of good physical health will normally produce adequate defences in response to infection, but deficiences in health, such as poor nutritional status, will impair that response.

Psychosocial Well-Being

The promotion of psychosocial well-being and the reduction of stress give maximum support to an individual's natural defence mechanisms. It has been suggested that stress may lower a person's resistance to infection (Ashworth, 1984) and further research needs to be undertaken in this important field.

Underlying Disease

The presence of underlying disease, such as pre-existing infection, diabetes, immune deficiency disease, vascular insufficiency, neoplasm or leukaemia, will render an individual more susceptible to infection.

Medical Intervention

Impaired resistance may arise as a direct result of treatment for a medical problem. The administration of antibiotics may alter normal body flora, while cancer chemotherapy, steroids and drugs to counteract organ transplant rejection interfere with immune mechanisms.

CATEGORIES OF HAI

Figure 4.2 shows the main types of HAI present in the UK.

Urinary Tract Infections

It is salient to realise that urinary tract infection (UTI) is the most common type of HAI and that three-quarters of UTI cases are found in patients who have undergone catheterisation. The 1980 HAI prevalence survey (Meers et al, 1981) showed that, of those patients with indwelling catheters, 21 per cent had a UTI whereas, of those without a catheter, only 3 per cent were infected. Catherisation is the most frequent cause of hospital infection and, in the above report, it was suggested that at least 500 people die each year in the UK as the result of urinary tract infection.

Wound Infection

When considering wound infection, it is important to establish the state of the

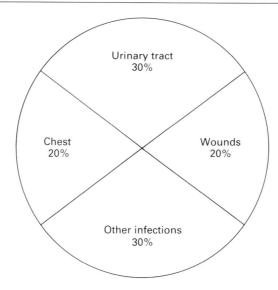

Fig 4.2 Categories of hospital-acquired infection in the UK

wound, as contaminated wounds are much more often infected than are clean ones. Reported wound infections rates vary from 20.6 per cent following gall bladder surgery to as little as 2.9 per cent following orthopaedic surgery (Imperial Chemical Industries, 1981). In Canada (Cruse, 1981) a study of 52 939 wound sites demonstrated a clean wound infection rate of 1.5 per cent and a dirty wound infection rate of 40 per cent. Infection in dirty wounds, i.e. where pus was found at the time of operation, was therefore more than 20 times higher than in clean wounds, a fact which has clear implications for nursing practice.

Chest Infection

Lower respiratory tract infections (LRTIs) are acquired almost twice as often in the community as they are in hospital. This is because sufferers from LRTI tend to be elderly with a history of chronic bronchitis and often have a variety of other contributory factors such as obesity or immobility. Upper respiratory tract infections (URTIs) are more likely to be seen in hospitals especially in paediatric and ENT wards.

Other Infections

This miscellaneous group includes any infection which does not come into one of the three preceding groups, e.g. those of skin, bones and joints, eyes, gastrointestinal tract, central nervous system, ears or circulation.

FACTORS ASSOCIATED WITH COMMUNITY ACQUIRED INFECTION

Patients in hospital are more vulnerable to infection than are those in the community. If people nursed in their own homes do not encounter similar infection risks to those who are nursed in hospital, what risks *do* they face in the community? Individual factors influencing powers of resistance will be common to both hospital and community patients but, once outside hospital, the general factors associated with acquired infection change.

Contact with Other People

A person at home will not usually come into contact with a large number of people. Far from being in close proximity to others, he is effectively isolated and will not be at risk from other patients or from staff who are sources or carriers of pathogens microbes.

Antibiotic-Resistant Microorganisms

Antibiotic-resistant strains of organisms are less likely to be found in the home, although it must be remembered that a patient at home with a chronic illness may be at risk from having received repeated antibiotic chemotherapy. A patient who is colonised or infected with an antibiotic-resistant bacterial strain may be both admitted from and discharged to his home, so the potential for microbial transfer between hospital and the community is always present.

Bypassing of Natural Defences

It is currently estimated that about 60 per cent of hospital-acquired infection is caused by Gram-negative organisms (Jenner and O'Neill, 1984) and, as these infections are usually associated with instrumentation or hospital equipment, the risk to the patient is considerably lessened if he stays at home. It is important, though, to be aware of the potential risk when bypassing the natural defence mechanisms in the home situation, e.g. during maintenance of total parenteral nutrition (TPN) or with continuous ambulatory peritoneal dialysis (CAPD).

A patient at home is often advantaged by being in a better general state of health than is a hospitalised patient. Seventy-eight per cent of patients seen at home are over 65 years of age (Jenner and O'Neill, 1984) and, as these people will, to some extent, demonstrate impairment of their defences towards infection, they will benefit from not being exposed to the hospital environment.

Trends in health care are encouraging shorter hospital stays, but this has the knock-on effect of increasing the number of potentially vulnerable people in the community, as well as of increasing the demand on community services.

THE CONSEQUENCES OF HOSPITAL-ACQUIRED INFECTION

Consequences for the Patient

At the very least, HAI complicates a person's recovery, increases his discomfort and prolongs his stay in hospital, on average by four days (Taylor, 1986). The results of sepsis range from the negligible effects of a small stitch abcess to death from septicaemia. Infection in a postoperative wound may impair the outcome of an operation or cause the wound to rupture, and infection after vascular surgery may necessitate limb amputation. An infected skin graft may fail to take. Certain types of infection may lead to disability, be it temporary or protracted, partial or complete.

A person with an infection will often suffer increased pain and undergo extra treatment. He will be anxious and may fail to maintain confidence in his carers. He will be further stressed if he is physically isolated from other patients on the ward. His family's concern will be an added burden to him, and he may be anxious about loss of earnings and job security. Such stresses adversely affect his powers of recovery.

Some of the more indirect consequences of hospital infection are difficult to assess, but it is clear that each prolonged stay in hospital means that another patient needing admission will have to wait a little longer. No estimate can be made of the increased discomfort and pressure that this can put on that person even before he has entered hospital.

Consequences for the Community

A patient may still carry a pathogenic organism after discharge from hospital. It has been demonstrated that patients harbouring antibiotic-resistant staphylococci at their time of discharge can continue to carry the strain for between six and 12 months, and that babies born in hospital may continue to harbour resistant staphylococci for longer periods after discharge than do adults (Verslagen et al, 1979).

Consequences for Hospital Staff

Hospital-acquired infection places an additional burden on the time and resources of a hospital and its personnel. When staff are busy, the pressure of the extra workload may become unacceptable, affecting the morale of nurses as well as of patients. Investigations into the source and nature of HAI further increase the throughput of work for laboratory staff.

HAI may result in concern and anguish for hospital personnel who have received inadequate information and instruction. Poorly informed staff who do not have a clear understanding of the situation may show a reluctance to work in an area where infection is present. Infection is historically associated with uncleanliness, and the stigma and fear of contracting an infection are very real concerns for many people.

Revenue Consequences

Combined expenses resulting from hospital-acquired infections are high. The total cost is difficult to assess and the very real costs of pain and suffering cannot be measured. Costing figures for HAI do not take into account loss of earnings, loss of productivity, loss of income tax, supplementary social security payments, the extra cost of treatment or the drain on priority services and those supporting delayed pre-admission patients. What can be measured is the cost of the extra days a patient spends in hospital as a result of HAI. In practice, these extra days represent a reduction in the number of beds available for patients on the waiting list. It is interesting to speculate then that the cost of these extra days does not necessarily represent actual increased cost to the hospital (Ayliffe et al, 1983).

It is known that:

- The mean 'hotel cost' of an acute hospital bed is £80 per day (DHSS/PHLS Hospital Infection Working Group, 1988)
- The average number of patients per bed per annum is 42 (Imperial Chemical Industries, 1981; cost calculation based on DHSS data)
- On average, four extra days are spent in hospital after infection has been acquired (DHSS/PHLS Hospital Infection Working Group, 1988)

Using these figures it is possible to estimate the hotel costs of infection for an acute unit. These costs cover hotel services only and are exclusive of the cost of treatments and specialist facilities.

Let us take, for example, an 'acute' hospital with 500 beds, each of which has 42 occupants in a year. A rate of infection of 5 per cent may be expected. (It should be noted that 5 per cent is expressed in the calculation as 5/100.)

The cost of extra days in hospital can be calculated using the following:

- Total number of patients × Infection rate (%) × Average number of extra days spent in hospital × Cost per day.

Using this formula:

Annual extra hotel cost	Total = number of patients	Infection × rate	Average × number of extra days in hospital	Cost × per day	
	= 21 000	× 5/100	× 4	× 80	= £33 600

Forty-five per cent of hospital beds in England and Wales are designated 'acute' (surgery, medicine, gynaecology, etc.). This results in the provision of 4.5 million acute beds. It is estimated that 90 000 beds are lost to HAI each year, and the hotel cost of these acute beds is estimated to be £76 million per annum. The potential saving from the prevention of HAI across the country can easily be imagined.

References

Ashworth P (1984) Infection control and the nursing process – making the best use of resources. *Journal of Hospital Infection*, **5**, supplement, pp. 35–44.

Ayliffe G A J, Collins B J and Taylor L J (1983) *Hospital Acquired Infection: Principles and Prevention*. Bristol: John Wright.

Cruse P (1981) *Aspects of Infection Control – Factors Influencing Surgical Wound Infections*. Macclesfield: ICI plc.

DHSS/PHLS Hospital Infection Working Group (1988) *Guidance on the Control of Infection in Hospitals* (The Cooke Report), HC (88) 33. London: HMSO.

Haley, R W, Culver D H, White J W, Morgan W M, Emori J G, Munn V P and Hooton T M (1985) The efficiency of infection surveillance and control programs in preventing nosocomial infections in US hospitals. *American Journal of Epidemiology*, **121**(2): 182–205.

Imperial Chemical Industries (1981) *The Cost of Hospital Infection*. Macclesfield: ICI plc.

Meers P D, Ayliffe G A J, Emerson A M, Leigh D A, Mayon-White R T, McKintosh C A and Stronge L J (1981) Report on the national survey on infection in hospitals. *Journal of Hospital Infection* **12**, supplement.

Further Reading

Antrobus M (1984) Infection control in hospital and the community. *Nursing*, **2**(23), supplement, pp. 4–7.

Ayliffe G A J and Collins B J (1982) *Aspects of Infection Control – Infection Control in United Kingdom*. Macclesfield: ICI plc.

Ayliffe G A J and Taylor L J (1984) *Infection Control Slide Library*. Macclesfield: ICI plc.

Gillman M and Andrews S (1984) Practical problems in the community. Infection control in hospital and the community. *Nursing*, **2**(23), supplement, pp. 1–4.

Imperial Chemical Industries (1983) *Breaking the Chain of Hospital Infection*. Macclesfield: ICI plc.

Lowbury E J L, Ayliffe G A J, Geddes A M and Williams J D (1981) *Control of Hospital Infection – A Practical Handbook*, 2nd edn. London: Chapman and Hall.

Meers P D and Stronge L J (1980) Urinary tract infection. *Nursing Times*, special supplement 7.

Jenner E A (1983) Identification of the infected patient – infection control in hospital and the community. *Nursing*, **2**(19), supplement, pp. 1–3.

Jenner E A and O'Neill P (1984) Infection control in hospital and the community. *Nursing*, **2**(27), supplement, pp. 1–7.

Taylor L J (1986) Hospital acquired infection. *Self Health*, **11**: 8–9.

Verslagen, Adviezen and Rapparten (1979) *Preventing Hospital Infections: Guidelines Proposed by the Health Council of the Netherlands*. Leidschendam, The Netherlands: Ministry of Health on Environmental Protection.

Weymont G (1984) Equipment and products. Infection control in hospital and the community. *Nursing*, **2**(24): 1–3.

5

The Control and Prevention of

Hospital-Acquired Infection

Infection will always be present somewhere in a hospital. The nurse's objective is to prevent its transmission to new hosts and new environments. The application of effective measures to control and prevent the spread of infection requires an understanding of how different microorganisms move around (see chapter 3). The answers to three questions are necessary to plan a strategy for preventing infection:

1. What is the source of infection?
2. Who or what is the susceptible host?
3. What is the means of transmission?

The **source of infection** can be reduced or removed by such measures as improved hospital design, treatment, discharge or isolation of the patient and disinfection or sterilisation of contaminated articles.

A **susceptible host** can be protected by means such as immunisation, sterilisation of objects with which he will come in to contact, transferring him out of a high-risk environment and not carrying out routine pre-operative shaving (Winfield, 1986).

The **means of transmission** can be restricted by, for instance, hand-washing, using disposable equipment, limiting staff movement and performing fewer invasive procedures.

Disruption of the method of spread arrests a microorganism's progress. If a person usually receives his salary in the form of a cheque sent through the mail, a postal strike will interrupt the normal channel for payment. In the same way, a microorganism that is denied its normal mode of spread will be thwarted in its aim of causing infection.

When fundamental microbial behaviour is understood, the control and prevention of infection becomes achievable. Successful control and prevention includes training for the carers, planning and organisation for the hospital, and effective management of both (table 5.1).

HEALTH-CARE WORKERS

Physicians, surgeons and nurses frequently appear to dismiss HAI as being of little importance or an inescapable accompaniment of hospital life (Worsley, 1983). This

Table 5.1   Factors influencing the prevention of infection

People

Immunity status	Training and education
Attitude and commitment	Personal hygiene
Presence of infection control personnel	

Environment

Building and design	Environment hygiene (cleaning, sterilisation,
Fixtures, fittings and furniture	laundry, catering, waste disposal)
Clinical equipment	Control of antibiotics and disinfectants
Hospital management	

attitude is unfortunate as the 1980 UK HAI prevalence survey (Meers et al, 1981) estimated that 50 per cent of HAI is preventable. Where multidisciplinary commitment to prevent and control infection replaces apathy there is enormous scope for success. In practice, this commitment is not easy to achieve because individuals select what they consider, or choose to consider, to be important and relevant.

The hospital service comprises many people practising a diversity of skills. To the domestic cleaner, having a patient in source isolation may mean the use of extra equipment, the application of specific cleaning practices and the perceived risk of taking the infection home to a young family. The doctor may see the same situation as being a nuisance, requiring only nurses to take protective measures.

Many health-care workers have a fear of acquiring an infection, so training and education needs to be given. Even then the unease may not be allayed completely. Such fear is often based on ignorance and the stigma associated with acquiring particular infections may also threaten credibility and status within the peer group. The belief that poor personal hygiene is associated with infection remains prevalent. Even when it is clear that this is not the reason for infection, it may be difficult to convince people of this truth.

Multidisciplinary training should share a common core of infection control knowledge. Thinking along similar lines should enable collaboration and promote co-operation with interdependent responsibilities. Compliance with infection control guidelines demonstrates professional competence but, unfortunately, there may remain a reluctance to work as normal in the face of a perceived risk and infected patients may, effectively, be ostracised. Florence Nightingale observed, 'Does not the popular idea of "infection" involve that people should take greater care of themselves than of the patient? That, for instance, it is not to be too much with the patient, not to attend too much of his wants?' (Nightingale, 1859).

Health-care workers have different jobs, different training needs and different standards of practice. There is no room, however, for different people to practise different control and prevention measures and specialist infection control personnel have a responsibility to lead the way in this important field.

Infection Control Personnel

In the UK, it is the responsibility of each health authority to ensure that the prevention and control of infection can be effectively practised. Most authorities discharge this duty through an infection control committee, the core of which is the infection control team. The functions and duties of the infection control service are illustrated in figure 5.1 (Lowbury et al, 1982).

Infection Control Committee

The function of this committee is to consider the overall strategy for and priorities in matters concerning the spread of infection. Health authority policies on disinfection and sterilisation, antibiotics, patient isolation, etc., will be referred to the committee. The committee members need to be aware of current infection surveillance studies and problems, and should be involved in the dissemination of infection control information.

The committee usually consists of a medical microbiologist, an infection control officer, an infection control nurse, representatives of the medical, nursing, pharmacy, central sterile supply department (CSSD), occupational and environmental health staff and the hospital administration. Heads of departments are co-opted onto the committee when the need arises.

Infection Control Officer

The infection control officer heading the infection control team should be a senior

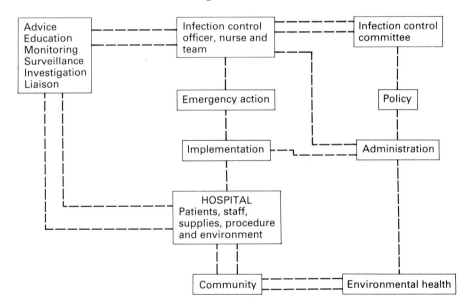

Fig 5.1   The Infection Control Service
(From Ayliffe and Collins, 1982. Reproduced by kind permission of ICI plc)

member of the medical staff with a special interest and training in infection control. In practice, 75 per cent of infection control officers in England and Wales are consultant microbiologists. He or she is responsible for identifying problems associated with infections or the risk of infection, and for advising on necessary control measures.

Infection Control Team

The minimum membership of the team is the infection control officer and infection control nurse but other medical and nursing staff, as well as scientific or technical staff specialising in infection control, may be included. The team takes responsibility for infection control both on a day-to-day and a long-term basis.

Infection Control Nurse

The infection control nurse (ICN) is usually the only full-time member of the infection control service. He or she is in daily contact with wards and departments. It is essential that good working relationships are established with all grades and all disciplines of health-care staff. It has been suggested (Walters, 1984) that, without a good sense of humour, an ICN will never acquire a balanced attitude. An ICN may be quizzed at any time by anyone on any aspect of infection control. Table 5.2 gives examples of questions such an ICN was asked during a salmonella outbreak.

While the ICN works with many people, maintenance of a close link with the occupational health nurse (OHN) is particularly advisable. Dialogue between these two disciplines is often symbiotic. Information given by one party often necessitates action by the other; for instance both will be involved when several nurses from the same residence report diarrhoea and vomiting, and follow-up will be required for contacts of a hospitalised patient with previously undiagnosed open pulmonary tuberculosis.

During an outbreak of infection the occupational health department plays an active role in the management of the situation. Ayton (1981) reports that, during an

Table 5.2   A sample of questions for an ICN during a salmonella outbreak

● Can salmonella-excreting employees attend a party in their hospital residence?	● What should be done about the salmonella-excreting patient who has discharged herself from hospital?
● Can residential salmonella-excreting staff use the staff canteen?	● An agency nurse's 10-month-old daughter has developed diarrhoea. What is the hospital's responsibility?
● Is a prison population at risk from a warden whose wife is a symptomatic hospital staff member?	● Can the infection control team guarantee that the domestic staff will not become salmonella excretors?
● As the asymptomatic domestic worker has been found to be a salmonella excretor, is it necessary to give time off to his asymptomatic domestic wife who works on a different ward?	● A salmonella-excreting patient has a daughter who works in a school canteen. Can this daughter take her mother's hospital clothes home to wash?
● What should the ambulance crew do about the patient from the hospital who has had a bout of diarrhoea in the ambulance?	● How should hospital laundry be handled now that the barrier-wash is malfunctioning?

outbreak of beta-haemolytic Lancefield Group A streptococci on a children's ward, the occupational health department prepared a record of all staff who had worked in the ward, contacted them, requested that they submit nose and throat swabs and gave subsequent advice on appropriate action and treatment.

Training and Education

Training for Hospital Staff

The ICN participates in education and training programmes on infection control for all health-care workers. The ICN herself needs specialist post-basic training and should have developed teaching skills. Newly appointed ICNs can attend a national orientation programme organised by the Infection Control Nurses Association (ICNA), and the English National Board (ENB) also runs infection control nursing courses.

ENB course no. 329 is a foundation course in infection control nursing for RGNs. It involves the study of infection control, the role and responsibilities of the infection control nurse, the hospital environment, microbiology and epidemiology, relationships and communication. ENB course no. 910 is a short update course open to RGNs who have been working in the field of infection control for at least three years. It aims to teach new developments and update and refresh skills and knowledge while also providing the opportunity to study different methods, policies and practices in relation to infection control.

The teaching and training of hospital staff will be formal or informal as appropriate. The effectiveness of informal teaching is sometimes underestimated as Gray (1986) reminds us:

● 'In former times, casual encounters of colleagues in hospital corridors and lunch-time table-talk probably did more for medical education than all the grandiose policy documents which nowadays are so common.'

To assist the ICN in her formal teaching role the ICNA has produced a wide range of audiovisual presentations covering major topics in infection control.

Educating Patients and Visitors

Hospital staff are not the only people needing guidance. Patients and relatives need to have infection control measures explained so that they, too, can help in care. Advice on arrangements for visitors will be required, especially for relatives visiting a patient in source isolation, who must receive clear instructions on self-protection measures. A patient with a highly communicable disease should not be visited by a susceptible person, but the nurse needs to explain why and define who a 'susceptible person' is (see chapters 3 and 4).

There is no evidence to show that visitors play a major role in hospital infection. As long as a visitor is healthy, follows hospital policy and does not return to an at-risk person or group in the community, there seems to be no valid reason to prohibit his visit. More importantly, a visit will usually be of enormous benefit to the patient.

In the interests of safety, visits by young children may need close supervision. There is the cautionary tale of the five-year-old who came with Mum to visit his sister in the special care baby unit. After his visit, no oxygen could be coaxed from the wall-mounted piped-oxygen ports. Other wards were not experiencing the same problem so the hospital engineer came to investigate. The mystery was solved when he extracted the rolled-up bus tickets which the little boy had forced into the outlet ports.

PERSONAL HYGIENE

Maintenance of personal hygiene is a part of everyday social and professional life to which we become accustomed from our early years. There is nothing technical or complicated about it, and it is incorporated into models of nursing as an activity of daily living. It must, however, be remembered that personal standards vary greatly.

In hospital surroundings, added precautions need to be taken. Health authorities should have a policy on uniform, and all hospital employees should be supplied with adequate changes of suitable clothing. This apparel should be laundered by the hospital and work clothing should be worn only in the hospital area.

Employees should be helped to understand that microorganisms that do not harm them could severely affect a susceptible host. The whitlow that is uncomfortable for the ancillary worker buttering the bread could be the potential cause of staphylococcal food poisoning for the patient. Any potential infection, skin lesion, rash, intestinal disturbance, sore throat or infected cut should be reported to the occupational health department.

The dispersal of resident skin staphylococci can be limited by such simple personal hygiene measures as bathing or showering, keeping nails short and unvarnished, keeping hair off, or tied back above, the collar and not wearing rings or other jewellery. It has been demonstrated that even the wearing of a wedding ring alters the natural skin flora, enabling potentially dangerous Gram-negative bacteria to colonise the skin underneath. In a study by Hoffman et al (1985), it was found that, following removal of a wedding ring, six weeks elapsed before normal skin flora were established. Earrings have the additional potential problem of being pulled and twisted by confused or paediatric patients.

The most important element in personal hygiene is hand-washing (see chapter 8). Taylor (1978) has observed an average hand-washing time of about 20 seconds among various grades of nurses, with individual times of between 5 and 120 seconds. Technique was usually found to be inadequate, with large areas of hand frequently left unwashed. Covert observation revealed that hands were often not washed at all after carrying out 'dirty' activities likely to leave them highly contaminated.

THE INFLUENCE OF THE ENVIRONMENT

The role of the environment in transferring infection is not always clear. To quote Collins (1981):

● 'A rotten apple in a barrel contaminating the rest has some similarities with a hospital. Failure to recognise a bad apple or to appreciate its importance when packing the barrel can initiate the problem. After this the size of the barrel and how full it is will determine the number of apples that can become bad. Checking the apples and removing bad ones may stop the process spreading and spraying or wrapping the apples or dividing the barrel into sections may reduce the number of casualties. The design of the barrel and how well it is maintained can also have some effect. However, failures in managing storage are usually more important. Complaining about the barrel without taking any other action will not save the apples.'

Design and Use of Space

People will always be the main factor in transmitting infection and a hospital's design should attempt to minimise this risk. Clean and dirty activities should be separate, allowing always for a flow of work from a clean to a dirty area.

An infected patient will contaminate most highly his immediate environment and disturbed pathogens will decrease in number with increasing distance from the patient. The risk of acquisition of illness is also related to the amount of time a person is close to the contaminated source, so the patient in the next bed will be most likely to acquire the infection, the nurse attending the patient is less likely to become ill and the rest of the staff attending the patient only infrequently are unlikely to become colonised or infected.

The Department of Health and Social Security hospital building note 4 (Department of Health and Social Security, 1968) gives details of floor space requirements. In an area providing a 30-bed nursing unit, it recommends 124 sq ft or 136 sq ft for a single room, 87 sq ft per bed for a multi-bed area and 18 sq ft per bed for a day space.

Building Maintenance

For infection control measures to be successful, it is necessary for the fabric of the building to be maintained to a high standard. In these days of economic stringencies, there are all too often insufficient funds to sustain rolling maintenance programmes. The missing ceiling tile, the split linoleum and the peeling wall paint will neither increase staff morale nor decrease the level of environmental microflora.

Air

Air is the one part of the environment that is shared by everyone and is in contact with everything. The number of organisms present in room air will depend on the number of people occupying the room, the degree of activity and the rate at which the air is replaced.

Most of these organisms will be Gram-positive cocci originating from the skin, with the potentially pathogenic *Staphylococcus aureus* accounting for less than 1 per cent of the total population. This is because staphylococci hitch-hike on skin scales which are heavy and cannot remain suspended for long. Droplets also do not travel easily, usually being carried only a few feet before they settle. Gram-negative bacteria are rarely found in the air because they die on drying and are thus dependent on aerosolisation.

The infection risk from open ward air is slight, and mechanical ventilation is not indicated. When source isolation is being practised, extract or negative pressure ventilation will ensure that air from the cubicle is extracted to the outside of the building. When protective isolation is in operation, the air coming into the room passes through a microbial filter before being delivered into the cubicle at positive pressure (figure 5.2).

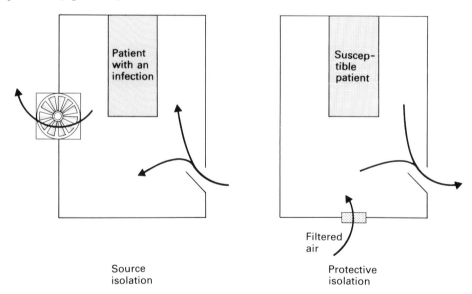

Fig 5.2   Airflow in source and protective isolation

In operating theatres, a system of 20 air changes per hour is usually used. Provision of complex ventilation systems, such as laminar flow or the Charnley method, may be justified when large incisions are kept open for long periods of time and where implants or transplants are involved. It has been suggested that halving the number of people in the operating theatre will probably halve the number of infections.

According to Cox (1977):

● 'A very potent way of churning up particles is to have the nurses around the theatre wearing skirts. As the skirt moves backwards and forwards there is a bellows action and "gulps" of air are formed which pick up particles and push them into the atmosphere. Even worse are stockings or tights which are marvellous ways of encouraging the skin scales to come off the skin; acting almost like cheese graters, they rub the skin particles off the legs, which are then picked up by the velocities and pushed into the atmosphere.'

For these reasons, nurses in operating theatres should always wear trousers.

Cox has also commented on typical face-masks. Schlieren photography, a specialised technique for identifying airflow patterns, has shown that quite high velocities of air at the sides of the face-mask are capable of picking up skin particles released both by the mask itself and by spectacles rubbing against the skin. This movement of air, along with that associated with breathing, is capable of disseminating particles into the atmosphere.

Flooring

Bacteria-laden particles will settle fairly rapidly onto horizontal surfaces, the most extensive of which is the floor. The number of bacteria present on the floor of a busy 30-bed ward can be quite high, maybe between 1000 and 2000 colony-forming units per 100 cm^2 (Ayliffe et al, 1984). Although the risk of infection from a hospital floor is slight for the mobile adult, it is much greater for the one-year-old who crawls everywhere and tests everything by taste.

About 99 per cent of organisms on a dry floor in a hospital ward are likely to be potentially non-pathogenic Gram-negative cocci. Despite this, these microorganisms and their attendant skin scales must be removed in order to maintain a safe environment. To permit their thorough cleaning, floors should have an impermeable hard covering without joints and with welded or sealed wall junctions.

The type and methods of maintenance of a carpet are important but there is no evidence that, providing a carpet is cleaned correctly, the infection risk will be any greater than that from a hard floor. The odour of stale urine often associated with hospital carpeting can be eradicated if carpet tiles are used and replaced as necessary.

Irrespective of the type of floor covering, some organisms will be able to survive if protected by layers of grease or protein from blood, urine or other secretions, so spillages and splashes should be wiped up immediately.

Walls and Ceilings

To minimise bacterial counts, walls should ideally have a smooth, hard, impervious, jointless, unbroken surface and be clean and dry; bacteria do not readily adhere to vertical surfaces or ceilings unless these are moist, sticky or damaged.

Paint used in operating theatres should be antistatic and expandable which will prevent cracks developing with changes in room temperature.

Fixtures and Fittings

The number of fixtures and fittings should be kept to an acceptable minimum, and they should be made from impervious material, without nooks and crannies where dirt or food particles can become trapped. Bacteria-laden particles easily settle on horizontal surfaces but cannot gain purchase on clean vertical or inverted surfaces. Surfaces should, therefore, be few, flat, easy to clean and unable to accumulate and retain dust and moisture.

Wash-Basins

Sinks and wash-basins should be sealed to the wall to allow proper cleaning, and splash-backs will help to prevent wall damage. Hand contact with taps should be avoided in clinical areas, and elbow-operated taps should be installed. As moisture-loving Gram-negative organisms commonly colonise 'U'-bends and sink outlets, the tap outflow should not point directly into the sink outlet; the subsequent splashing could disperse contaminated aerosols from a colonised trap or 'U'-bend.

Trapped bacteria are present around the sink outlet and will be resuspended in the water if the sink is filled, so hand-washing should be performed in running water. Plugs ought not to be provided as their use in clinical areas allows the filling of a dirty sink, with a resultant wash in a bacterial soup.

Sink overflow outlets should be avoided as they are difficult to clean and become colonised with Gram-negative bacteria.

Furniture

All furniture should be readily cleanable, have an impervious finish and be free from ledges. Manufacturers should provide users with details of suitable cleaning and decontamination methods to enable furniture to be kept free from bacteria-supporting soil.

The importance of cleanliness of furniture can be shown by the following by the following unpublished example of a methicillin resistant *Staphylococcus aureus* (MRSA) problem in a ward caring for the elderly. Despite stringent control measures, perineal MRSA colonisation recurred in two patients. On closer examination it was found that these people, who spent much of their day out of bed, had not once had their wheelchairs washed. Although no MRSA-positive cultures were obtained from the wheelchairs, the problem resolved when daily wheelchair cleaning was commenced.

Bedding

Mattresses and pillows should have impervious covers, and it should be remembered that some plastics become permeable when repeatedly subjected to certain disinfectants. This may allow colonisation of the interior of the mattress or pillow. If waterproof covers on pillows are not acceptable to the patient, a suitable method for cleaning the pillow must be available. Duvets are being increasingly used in geriatric, psychiatric and mental illness areas, and must be fire-retardant and washable.

CLINICAL EQUIPMENT

Quality control of all hospital equipment should minimise risk to patients. False economy will often result from selecting the cheapest item available, as it may not function adequately; twice as much adhesive tape may be required to make the dressing stick; two paper towels may have to be used instead of one; the arthritic patient may be unable to operate the tap of a particular urinary drainage bag.

All hospital equipment needs to conform to the British Standards Institute or Department of Health specifications, fire and safety regulations and professional criteria. In the UK, a 'Guide to Good Manufacturing Practice for Sterile and Medical Devices and Surgical Products' (see Hardie, 1982) covers the basic concepts and principles of good manufacturing practice. The DHSS register contains only the names of approved manufacturers of sterile medical devices and surgical products, and the Department of Health circulates equipment hazard notices as appropriate. These should be acted on and not merely filed away.

Many district and regional health authorities now have their own policies for co-ordinating equipment trials. Such trials should never be negotiated with a visiting salesman. One ICN discovered to her surprise that a company representative had furnished five of the hospital wards with urinary draining bags, penile sheaths and equipment questionnaires. This was strange because the hospital was not conversant with the firm, but stranger still because three of the wards housed female patients only.

Disposable Items

When disposable items were first introduced, it was suggested that infection risks from equipment would be virtually eliminated (Causier, 1982) and that savings would be made in manpower and machinery as recycling would become unnecessary. In practice, hospitals cannot afford, store or dispose of all these items (figure 5.3) and re-use of some disposable items often occurs. Manufacturers, however, will not accept responsibity for the performance of recycled items, so the use of such products needs to be carefully monitored.

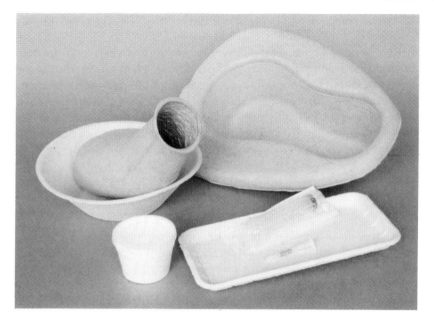

Fig 5.3   The proliferation of disposal articles

Medical Equipment

In the UK, we rely on complex medical equipment to diagnose, treat and monitor patients (Collins, 1982a). The equipment often includes electronic components, fibreoptic bundles, plastics and other heat-sensitive items. In the surgical field, anaesthetic and respiratory equipment and endoscopes are frequently used.

To minimise the risk of infection, there must be facilities available to decontaminate adequately all clinical equipment. Hospitals with a medical equipment cleaning department (MED) can ensure that the health authority protocol is followed, provide a central pool of equipment and supply trained engineering staff. It is possible to process a limited amount of medical equipment through central sterile supply departments (CSSDs) and theatre sterile supplies units (TSSUs).

Installation and Maintenance of Equipment

Equipment should be correctly installed and, thereafter, be properly maintained. A common example of shortfall in this area is the humble bedpan washer/disinfector. The machine disinfects by raising the temperature of the bedpan to a minimum of 80°C for one minute by using steam during the final stage of the cleaning cycle. Very often, checks will reveal that such equipment is not working adequately.

A 1976 survey by Dorning correlated information on bedpan washers from 60 infection control nurses. Common faults mentioned were poor water pressure, blockage by solids, attachment to wrong-size pipes, inadequate drainage and low water levels in the tanks. Maintenance was sometimes made difficult due to insufficient space left at the side of the machine for access to working parts and many machines had not been installed by the manufacturers, but, rather, by contractors or local engineers (Dorning, 1976).

Of the 1050 washers surveyed, one third were generally unreliable. Dorning also found that nurses tended not to use the bedpan washers, and it was estimated that at any one time about half of the machines were malfunctioning.

Bedpan macerators used for the disposal of matter other than human exudate will also break down, and aerosolisation of macerator contents will occur if the seal on the lid is not air-tight. As well as posing a health hazard, such inefficient equipment also leads to wasteful expenditure.

HOSPITAL HYGIENE

Cleaning

Dirt is multi-talented: it corrodes, abrades, reacts with chemicals, blocks channels, encourages pests, prevents disinfection and sterilisation and provides nutrients for microorganisms. The main methods of removing dirt are wet and dry cleaning, and the method of cleaning substantially influences airborne bacterial counts (table 5.3).

Table 5.3   Changes in airborne bacterial counts with different methods of cleaning floors

Method used	Change in bacterial count
Sweeping with broom	700% increase
Vacuum cleaning	20% decrease
Dust-attracting floor mop	30% increase
Wet scrubbing machine	3% increase

The effect may vary with the make of equipment and method of use

(From Ayliffe et al, 1983. Reproduced by kind permission of John Wright and Sons.)

Dry Cleaning

Even when used with care, brooms and brushes redisperse bacteria-laden particles into the air, and this dispersed dust then resettles. Dry mops used in hospitals should be specially treated to attract and retain dust particles.

Vacuum cleaning should increase airborne bacterial counts to a lesser extent than dry mopping, provided that the exhaust air is filtered and does not discharge dust into uncleaned areas.

High-dusting should be carried out with a vacuum head or a dust-retaining mop to prevent dust cascading onto the patient. In the days when high-dusting was performed with the aid of a piece of lint wrapped round a broom head, not only did the dust fly but also minute particles of lint were released with it (Brooke, 1977). In 1854, Florence Nightingale wryly observed, 'Dusting in these days means nothing but flapping the dust from one part of the room to another . . . what you do it for I cannot think.' (Nightingale, 1859)

Wet Cleaning

Dispersal of microorganisms into the air is less likely during wet cleaning than during dry cleaning. The most common and efficient wet cleaning solution used in hospitals is one of hot water and detergent which emulsifies the protein coat protecting the bacterial soil. The wash should be followed by rinsing to prevent the build-up of a detergent film, and this should be followed by drying. The cleaning equipment, too, must be rinsed and stored dry, and mop heads should be regularly processed by a laundry or central sterile supply department.

Cleaning of Isolation Cubicles

The correct procedure for cleaning isolation areas needs to be understood by the domestic staff, who also need to be aware of any potential risk to themselves or others. Clearly marked and separately stored equipment should be reserved for use in such areas. Disposable cloths should be used, and cleaning equipment kept to a minimum. Local health authority terminal cleaning methods must be followed on discharge of the patient.

Washing and Sanitary Facilities

Sink outlets, traps and overflows, drains, toilets and sluices are all likely to be heavily contaminated with Gram-negative bacteria. Disinfectants are of little value and may corrode pipes. When bleach is poured down a toilet, the next person who comes along flushes it away; Maurer (1985) points out that flushing the lavatory is more effective for reducing the numbers of microorganisms than is the addition of a chemical disinfectant.

When a patient has a bath, he shares it with millions of bacteria from his own skin and gut, to say nothing of those remaining from the previous person. Using a shower exposes a person to a lesser risk of cross-infection than does using a bath.

A bed-bound patient should be supplied with his own wash-bowl which should be stored dry and inverted, ideally in or at the back of the bedside locker. Greaves (1985), in a spot-check of wards, showed that, of 123 bowls in use, only 42 (34 per cent) had been thoroughly dried before storage (figure 5.4). In follow-up work, Beaker and Dealey (1986) found that only five nurses out of 27 had read Greaves' article and that none of the four wards she investigated had an explicit policy on wash-bowls. Another such survey, conducted on three wards (Hill, 1982) showed that only one nurse was found to be using the recommended cleaning agent for wash-bowls – general purpose detergent.

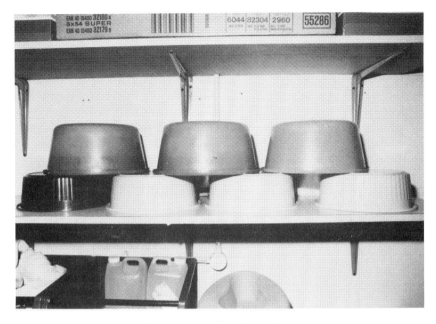

Fig 5.4   Correct storage of wash-bowls on the ward

Laundering

Department of Health and Social Security recommendations (1987) state that laundry should be divided into three categories:

1. Used (soiled and fouled)
2. Infected
3. Heat-labile

Linen is only considered infected if it has been used by patients with, or suspected of suffering from, enteric fever and other salmonella infections, dysentery (shigella species), hepatitis A and B (and hepatitis carriers), open pulmonary tuberculosis, human immunodefiency virus, notifiable diseases (see chapter 9) and other infections specified by the infection control officer as hazardous to staff. Linen in this category should not be sorted but be placed directly in a water-soluble bag which is sealed and placed in a red laundry bag.

A national colour code for identification of linen bags and containers is recommended:

● Used (soiled and fouled) – white
● Infected – red; this should carry a prominent yellow label such as 'Infected Linen'
● Heat-labile – white with a prominent orange stripe

A covered, dry holding area should house dirty linen prior to its collection. Laundry design should incorporate a separate loading area housing a machine designated for foul and infected linen.

All foreign objects must be removed from the linen before it is bagged to prevent harm to laundry workers and machines. Table 5.4 lists the items one health authority retrieved during one 12-week period.

All linen is heat disinfected at a temperature of 65°C for 10 minutes or 71°C for 3 minutes. Linen from a patient with hepatitis B is required to reach a minimum temperature of 95°C for 10 minutes. The provision of a barrier between the section which receives the 'used or infected' linen and the rest of the laundry is not considered necessary. It is recommended that 'infected' linen should be washed in a designated washer extractor. Domestic washing machines are used in some hospital areas. They pose little risk except during outbreaks of infection, when the temperature of the wash may need to be raised.

Catering

In February 1987, Crown Immunity from prosecution was withdrawn from UK hospitals. As a result, one area under noticeable scrutiny is the hospital kitchen where the correct storage and handling of food is now statutory.

Attention should be paid to the health of the catering staff both before taking up employment and during their tenure. Medical screening should be used to investigate histories of gastrointestinal illness, tuberculosis, skin rashes, etc.

High standards and correct methods of cleaning are essential in the catering department. Cleaned impervious surfaces should always be dry before use. Surfaces should be used for one purpose only and must be cleaned with a disposable cloth.

Table 5.4   Items retrieved from a health authority laundry during a 12-week period

1 screw	3 towel clips
1 nail	1 pair of curved scissors
1 tube of toothpaste	1 tongue clip
1 razor with blade	1 cord cutter
1 colour photograph	1 gate clip
1 set of upper and lower false teeth	2 curved artery forceps
1 set of upper false teeth	1 set of straight artery forceps
9 pairs of spectacles	1 bodkin
3 glass baby-feeding bottles (2 broken)	1 pair of dissecting forceps
3 hearing-aid ear-pieces	1 pair of long artery forceps
1 ball-point pen	1 sigmoidoscope attachment
1 shaving soap stick	1 connector for a sphygmomanometer
1 brass nut	1 metal X-ray marker
2 wrist watches	1 scalpel blade
2 keys with chain and fob	1 i.v. air inlet
Several metal paper fasteners	1 metal extension strap retainer
1 key	1 roll of dressing adhesive
13 name badges	1 cord clamp
1 pair of plastic tweezers	1 spinal needle
1 RCN badge	1 plug fuse
1 NUPE badge	1 wedding ring
1 radiographer's badge	1 handbag – recovered after it had been
1 cuff inflator	laundered
1 sphygmomanometer cuff	

In the kitchen heat is an effective infection control measure. Any food capable of supporting bacterial life should be stored below 6°C which will prevent the multiplication of most bacteria, or above 65°C. Any surface which has reached 65°C and is maintained at that temperature for 10 minutes, or has reached 80°C for a few seconds, is unlikely to be heavily contaminated with vegetative organisms. Cooked food which requires cooling should be placed in a designated 'rapid cool area' to reduce the food temperature from 70°C to 3°C in 1½ hours or less. Hot food transported to the wards in heated trolleys should be at a minimum temperature of 63°C before starting its journey, and it is advisable for thermometers to be incorporated into food trolleys.

'Cook–Chill' meal systems are often used and involve food being cooked, chilled and stored at or below 3°C. Food should not be kept for more than five days between cooking and consumption.

Crockery and cutlery should, ideally, be processed in a central washing-up machine at a minimum temperature of 60°C, the final rinse being at a minimum temperature of 82°C.

In the UK in 1984, there was a major outbreak of salmonella food poisoning in a hospital for mentally ill and psychogeriatric patients. Altogether 355 patients and 106 members of staff were affected, with food poisoning causing, or contributing to, the deaths of 19 patients (Department of Health and Social Security, 1986). The enquiry committee concluded that the cause of the outbreak was salmonella, which was probably brought into the kitchen in contaminated chickens and had then spread to other food-stuffs. Cold beef was the most likely vehicle and had become infected because it had not been properly refrigerated.

In a 1981–1982 prospective study in hospitals in England and Wales, 55 salmonella outbreaks were identified, but in only six (11 per cent) was food thought to be the source of infection (Cruickshank, 1984), and person-to-person spread was found to be the most important factor. It should be borne in mind that spread of infection is always possible by vehicles other than food or hands.

Disposal of Waste

A hospital's by-product is waste. In 1982 in England, Scotland and Wales, it was estimated (Murrell, 1982) that rubbish was produced at the rate of 4 lbs per bed per day (see also figure 5.5). Waste must be contained in colour-coded bags in accordance with local health authority policy. The Health Services Advisory Committee (1982) recommends the following colour-coding for containers holding clinical waste:

- Black – normal household waste; not to be used to store or transport clinical waste
- Yellow – waste destinated for incineration
- Yellow with a black band – waste (e.g. home nursing waste) which preferably should be disposed of by incineration but which may be disposed of by landfill, in which case separate collection and disposal arrangements should be made

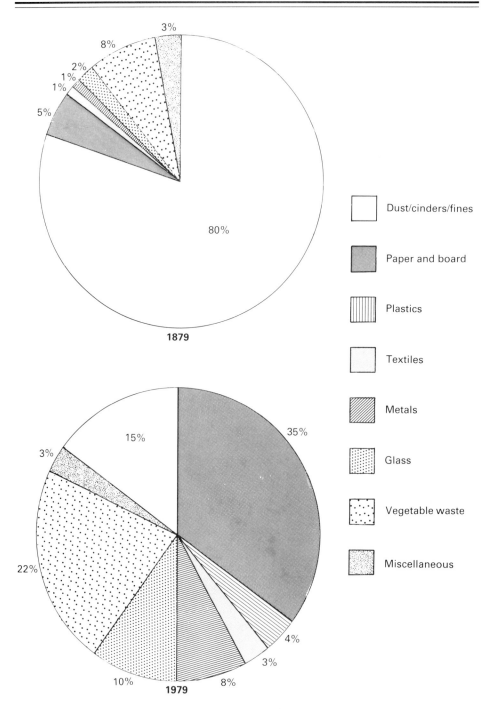

Fig 5.5   The increase in the disposal of waste

● Light blue or transparent with light blue inscriptions – waste for autoclaving (or equivalent treatment) before ultimate disposal

High-risk medical waste is autoclaved before being incinerated. Waste awaiting collection must be housed in a secure, washable, covered area to discourage attention from feral cats, rodents, children and drug users. All clinical waste should be incinerated and, in the community, arrangements need to be made for the collection of such material.

Disposal of Excreta

An ordinary bedpan washer/disinfector incorporating steam held at 80°C for one minute will disinfect. The steam, however, will not be effective unless all soil is first removed.

Bedpans or urinals used by patients with pathogenic enteric bacteria should be immediately disinfected in the bedpan disinfector. Covering the faeces with a chemical disinfectant and leaving them to soak is unnecessary, and the stool protein may inactivate the disinfectant before it fully penetrates the excreta. The disinfectant also increases the risk of bedpan content spillage.

Disposable papier-maché bedpans or urinals and their contents are disposed of in a macerator. The outer plastic bedpan holders must be kept soil-free by washing them with detergent and hot water and by ensuring that they are completely dry before their next use. In the absence of disinfectors or macerators, bedpans and urinals can be soaked in 1 per cent phenolic for 20 to 30 minutes.

Disposal of Sharp Instruments

Containers for used needles and sharp instruments ('sharps') must meet the nine criteria laid down in the DHSS specification (Department of Health and Social Security, 1982). All used disposable sharps must immediately be placed in a puncture-proof container, suitable for incineration, which must not be overfilled (figure 5.6). Approximately 40 per cent of self-inoculation accidents occur while resheathing needles (Advisory Committee on Dangerous Pathogens, 1986), so this must not be done unless there is a safe means available. Any accidental inoculation or cut involving needles or sharp instruments should be dealt with in accordance with the local health authority policy.

CONTROL OF ANTIBIOTICS

Antibiotic usage (see chapter 7) should be controlled as this will help to prevent the 'selecting out' of antibiotic-resistant organisms after antibiotic treatment has killed those which are sensitive. Following relevant consultation, primarily between the pharmacist and microbiologist, details of antibiotics routinely dispensed by a hospital pharmacy should be published.

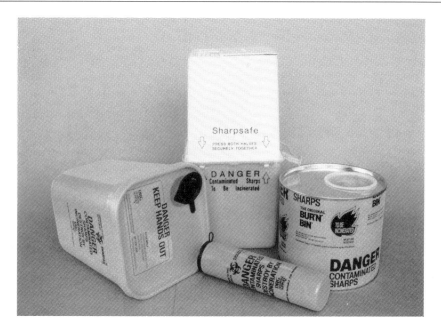

Fig 5.6   Containers used for the disposal of 'sharps'

DISINFECTION AND STERILISATION

There are three ways of removing or destroying microorganisms but these methods are not equally effective.

- *Cleaning* is the removal of dirt and many of the microorganisms present.
- *Disinfection* is the removal or destruction of microorganisms, not usually including bacterial spores which can be highly resistant to disinfection.
- *Sterilisation* is the removal or destruction of all microorganisms. This is an absolute condition: 'almost' and 'nearly sterile' are meaningless terms.

Cleaning should, if possible, be the first part of the disinfection and sterilisation process. Thorough cleaning with hot water and detergent removes both microorganisms and the dirt which can form a protective barrier around them.

Disinfection

Disinfection can be achieved by:

- Cleaning
- Heat
- Chemical solutions

These methods can be combined; e.g. dishwashers, washing machines and bedpan washer/pasteurisers remove the majority of microorganisms by cleaning, and then kill most of those remaining with heat.

Heat Disinfection

Disinfection by heat is always the method of choice. It is rapid, cheap and does not suffer from the many drawbacks that chemical disinfection does. Heat disinfection is one of the oldest techniques in microbiology and takes its name, **pasteurisation**, from Louis Pasteur, the nineteenth-century scientist who introduced it. It is still widely used today to ensure that milk is free from pathogenic microbes.

Heating liquids or immersing instruments in hot water is a reliable method of killing microorganisms other than bacterial spores. Disinfection temperatures and times range from 60°C for 10 minutes to 80°C or above for one minute, although extra time must be allowed for cold instruments to reach the disinfection temperature. This process is usually carried out in a hot water disinfector, sometimes wrongly called a boiling water steriliser: boiling water is not hot enough to sterilise.

Chemical Disinfection

Chemical disinfectants suffer from many drawbacks (table 5.5). Where conditions are ideal, especially in laboratory tests, some can be shown to sterilise, but these ideal conditions rarely occur in practice.

Some chemicals are sold as 'sterilants'. In laboratory tests they can produce sterility after, for example, three hours' contact time in the absence of dirt but, because they are called sterilants, some people will expect them to kill all microorganisms present in any situation. Soaking a soiled instrument in a sterilant for a minute or two does not lead to its sterilisation. It is best to think of sterilants as high-level disinfectants (when used properly), and not as a substitute for sterilisation by a more certain method (see below).

There are many disinfectants on the market and each one belongs to a chemical family with its own patterns of behaviour and range of activity. To know the characteristics of a particular brand of disinfectant, the chemical group to which it belongs must be known. Table 5.6 gives a summary of these groups and their characteristics.

Table 5.5   Factors affecting the efficacy of disinfectants

- Microbial challenge (numbers and types of organism)
- Disinfectant concentration
- Shelf life and use of life, i.e. length of active life once opened
- Dilution during use
- Pollution during use with inactivating substances
- Contact with inactivating substances, such as
    organic matter: food, faeces, blood, vomit, etc.
    soaps, detergents and other disinfectants
    hard water
    natural and synthetic materials: cork, rubber, cellulose and various plastics

Table 5.6 Summary of disinfectant groups

Group	Examples	Activity against: Bacteria	Spores	Viruses	Resistance to inactivation	Use	Remarks
Phenolic	Hycolin Stericol Izal	+	−	±	±	Environment	
Hypochlorite (bleach)	Milton Sterite Presept	+	±	+	−	Environment Equipment	Corrosive to metals. Causes irreparable damage to blood capillaries
Chlorhexidine	Hibitane Hibiscrub	+	−	±	−	Skin	Corrosive to tissue Is inflammable
Alcohol	Ethanol Isopropanol	+	−	+	+	Skin Surfaces	
Iodine	Aqueous iodine Tincture of iodine Betadine Disadine	+	±	+	−	Skin	Aqueous and tincture forms can cause irritation. May damage capillaries
Hexachlorophane	Ster-Zac	+	−	±	−	Skin	Caution with repeated use of emulsion in neonates
Triclosan	Manusept Cidal	+,	−	±	−	Skin	
Glutaraldehyde	Cidex Asep Totacide	+	+	+	+	Instruments	Irritating vapour
Quaternary ammonium compounds	Roccal Zephiran Cetavlon Dettox	+	−	±	−	Instruments Skin	Contamination problems; use with caution

Hospitals should have a disinfectant policy and a list of disinfectants and the purposes for which they can be used. This enables a hospital or health authority to buy disinfectants rationally and hospital staff to use them effectively. Irrational use of disinfectants is commonplace. Ward (1985) conducted a survey prior to the introduction of a particular health authority's disinfectant policy and found that nine different products were used for cleaning baths, showers and bowls, part of a long and confusing range of products used within the health authority. Thirty-three products, either disinfectants or containing a disinfectant agent, were identified, together with 24 cleaning agents.

Most disinfectants can, instead of killing bacteria, become colonised with them. This tends to happen when disinfectants have been inactivated in some way, have been in use too long or have not been made up to the correct dilution (see table 5.5).

For a disinfectant to be effective, the following principles should be followed:

- Choose the right disinfectant for the situation
- Use it at the appropriate strength
- Avoid diluting or polluting the disinfectant
- Allow sufficient contact time for it to act

Sterilisation

Sterilisation can be achieved by heat, irradiation or filtration.

Heat Sterilisation

Conditions for heat sterilisation can be either wet or dry. Steam transfers its heat far better than does air; steam from a kettle (at 100°C) will burn skin far more readily than air from a hot oven (at about 150°C). Sterilisation by steam takes place in an autoclave, which works by the same principle as a pressure cooker. Boiling water (100°C) is hot enough only to disinfect, but increasing the pressure in a container will enable boiling water and its steam to exist at temperatures above 100°C, where even bacterial spores can be killed. Sterilisation times and temperatures in an autoclave range from 15 minutes at 121°C to three minutes at 134°C.

Sterilisation by dry heat takes longer and uses higher temperatures (160°C for one hour is a common time and temperature combination), so only objects that are very heat resistant can be put through this process.

Irradiation

Sterilisation by irradiation is a very expensive system to set up and run, so is usually only used by manufacturers who can constantly feed production line items through an irradiation plant. The radiation dose normally given to ensure sterility is 2.5 megarads.

Filtration

Filtration is used to sterilise heat-sensitive solutions such as those used in total parenteral nutrition. A filter with pore size of 0.2 μm will remove all bacteria from a solution.

The degree of sterilisation or disinfection required in a given situation depends on the risk posed to the patient and may be classified as follows:

1. *High*   For equipment introduced into a sterile body area (surgical instruments, syringes, needles, etc.) or in close contact with a break in the skin. Sterilisation is usually required in this situation.

2. *Intermediate*   For equipment in close contact with body surfaces (respiratory apparatus, gastroscopes, bedpans, urinals, etc.). These usually require disinfection although cleaning may be adequate; a combination of both is usually recommended.

3. *Low* For the environment or equipment not in close contact with the patient (walls, floors, sinks, drains, etc.). Cleaning is usually adequate but in high risk units, such as operating theatres and isolation units, disinfection can be carried out.

INFECTION CONTROL POLICIES AND GUIDELINES

The principles of nursing are standard but their application is not, so assessment of a patient will produce an individualised care plan. So it is with infection control guidelines and policies: infection control principles are constant but the variables of health authorities are not, and local policy should reflect local circumstances and resources. Health authorities usually document their guidelines and policies in an infection control manual or book, which should be available to all health authority personnel.

Carers Outside Hospital

People other than health authority employees will also be concerned with infection control. When a patient with an infection is discharged to his home, questions are raised for local authority employees: social workers may enquire whether or not it is necessary to use protective clothing; home helps may be anxious about taking the infection into their own homes. 'Meals-on-wheels' volunteers may express concern about taking money from a client, while mobile library personnel may ask about the risk of infection from books which are returned to them. It often falls to the infection control nurse to field these questions and give reassurance.

Some disciplines, such as ambulance service workers, prepare their own regulations. All people requiring ambulance transport are categorised for infection risk, and the ambulance crew implement the control and disinfection measures relevant to the patient's category. In special circumstances, extra precautions may become necessary, such as during the 1985–86 methicillin-resistant *Staphylococcus aureus* (MRSA) outbreak in North London when comprehensive patient information had to be given before a patient with MRSA could be transported by ambulance.

SUMMARY

The task of preventing and controlling infection may appear Herculean, but most effective control measures are simple. Missionary zeal may result in wasted time spent collecting meaningless information; routine slit sampling of the operating theatre air, for example, will not further the control and prevention of infection.

Routine sampling is not usually justified, although, during an outbreak, screening of the staff and environment may be part of the control programme. Infection control measures should be relevant and uncomplicated. The health authority, through good management, should make the provision and co-ordination of all control measures possible.

Hand-washing remains the single most effective and economical means of controlling infection. Every health authority employee is responsible for his or her personal hygiene and standards of hand-washing. It must be remembered that, for both individual and health authority, control measures will only be as effective as their standard of application.

References

Advisory Committee on Dangerous Pathogens (ACDP) (1986) *LAV/HTLV III, The Causative Agent of AIDS and Related Conditions – Revised Guidelines*. London: DHSS.

Ayliffe G A J, Coates D and Hoffman P N (1984) *Chemical Disinfection in Hospitals*. London: Public Health Laboratory Services.

Ayliffe G A J, Collins B J and Taylor L T J (1983) *Hospital Acquired Infection: Principles and Prevention*. Bristol: John Wright.

Ayres D C (1982) *Disposal of Hospital and Domestic Waste and Land Reclamation*. Paper presented at the 13th Infection Control Nurses Association Symposium.

Ayton M (1981) An outbreak of streptococcal infection in a children's ward. *Nursing Times, Journal of Infection Control*, pp. 4–7.

Beaker M and Dealey C (1986) Actions speak louder than words. *Nursing Times*, **82**(20): 37–39.

Brooke (1977) *The Cleaning of our Hospitals*. Paper presented at the Infection Control Nurses Association Annual Conference 1977.

Causier P M (1982) The equipment resource. *Nursing*, **2**(8): 237–238.

Collins B J (1981) Infection and the hospital environment. *Nursing*, **29**(9): 1–3.

Collins B J (1982a) Medical equipment. *Nursing*, **2**(8): 233–234.

Collins B J (1982b) The use of chemical disinfectants in hospital. *Nursing*, **2**(7): 190–193.

Cox R N (1977) *The Human Micro-Environment*. Paper presented at the Infection Control Nurses Association Annual Conference 1977.

Cruickshank J G (1984) The investigation of salmonella outbreaks in hospitals. *Journal of Hospital Infection*, **5**(3): 241–243.

Department of Health and Social Security (1968) *Hospital Building Note 4 – Ward Units*. London: HMSO.

Department of Health and Social Security (Welsh Office) (1971) *Hospital Laundry Arrangements*. London: HMSO.

Department of Health and Social Security (1980) *Guidelines on Pre-cooked Chilled Foods*. London: HMSO.

Department of Health and Social Security (1982) *Specification for Containers for the Disposal of Used Needles and Sharp Instruments*. London: HMSO.

Department of Health and Social Security (1984) *The Report of the Committee of Enquiry into an Outbreak of Food Poisoning at Stanley Royd Hospital*. Chairman: Hughill J. London: HMSO.

Department of Health and Social Security (1987) *Hospital Laundry Arrangements for Used and Infected Linen*. London: HMSO.

Gray J (1986) Controlling infections – how well do we do it? *Journal of Infection*, **12**(3): 195–197.

Greaves A (1985) 'We'll just freshen you up, dear . . .' *Nursing Times* **81**(10), *Journal of Infection Control Nursing*, pp. 3–8.

Hardie I D (1982) Manufacture and irradiation sterilisation of sterile medical products. *Nursing*, **2(8)**: 223–225.

The Health Service Advisory Committee (HSAC) (1982) *The Safe Disposal of Clinical Waste*. London: HMSO.

Hill S (1984) Which disinfectants do nurses use? *Nursing Times*, **80**(7), *Journal of Infection Control Nursing*, pp. 60–61.

Hoffman P N, Cook E M, McCarville M and Emmerson A M (1985) Micro-organisms isolated from under wedding rings worn by hospital staff. *British Medical Journal*, **290**: 206–207.

Lowbury E J L, Ayliffe G A J, Geddes A M and Williams J D (1982) *Control of Hospital Infection: A Practical Handbook*, 2nd edn. London: Chapman and Hall.

Maurer I (1985) *Hospital Hygiene*, 3rd edn. London: Edward Arnold.

Meers P D, Ayliffe G A F, Emmerson A M, Leigh D A, Mayon-White R T, Mckintosh C A and Stronge L J (1981) Report of the National Survey on Infection in Hospitals. *Journals of Hospital Infection*, supplement 2.

Murrell H (1982) *Hazards and Policies of Hospital Waste*. Paper presented at the 13th Infection Control Nurses Association Symposium.

Nightingale F (1859) *Notes on Nursing what it is and what it is not*. Reprinted by Churchill Livingstone, Edinburgh, 1980.

Taylor L J (1978) An evaluation of handwashing techniques, I and II. *Nursing Times*, **74**(2): 54, **74**(3): 108–110.

Walters E M (1984) Disinfection and sterilisation. Infection control in hospital and the community. *Nursing*, **2**(24): 3–4.

Ward K (1985) Down the drain? *Nursing Times*, **81**(49), *Journal of Infection Control Nursing*, pp. 60–62.

Winfield N (1986) Too close a shave? *Nursing Times*, **82**(10), *Journal of Infection Control Nursing*, pp. 64–68.

Worsley M A (1983) *Guidance for Hospital Personnel*. A seminar on the control of hospital acquired infection. London: Update Publications.

Further Reading

Baxter B (1987) Too good to throw away. *Nursing Times*, **83**(11): 24–26.

Collins B J (1986) Respiratory assistance – care of equipment. *Intensive Care Nursing*, **1**: 138–143.

Department of Health and Social Security (1982) *Code of Practice for the Prevention of Infection in Clinical Laboratories and Post Mortem Rooms*. Chairman: Howie J. London: HMSO.

Department of Health and Social Security (1985) *Clean Catering – A Handbook on Hygiene in Catering Establishments*. London: HMSO.

Fletcher M K (1981) The role of nursing and medical staff in the prevention of hospital acquired infection. *Nursing*, **29**: 6–7.

Haley R W, Culver D H, White J W, Morgan W M, Emori J G, Munn V P and Hooton T M (1985) The efficacy of infection surveillance and control programmes in preventing nosocomial infections in US hospitals. *American Journal of Epidemiology*, **121**(2): 182–205.

Henderson M (1980) *Team up to Infection Control*. Paper presented at the Infection Control Nurses Association Annual Conference 1980.

Hoffman P N (1982) *Transient Contamination of Hands*. Paper presented at the 13th Annual Infection Control Nurses Association Symposium.

Hoffman P N (1986) Disinfection in hospitals. *Nursing*, **3**(3): 106–108.

Hunter I (1987) Is re-use worth the risk? *Nursing Times*, 29–30.

Jenner E A (1984) Under control. *Senior Nurse*, **1**: 14–16.

King Edward's Hospital Fund for London (1986) *Re-use of Sterile, Single Use and Disposable Equipment in the NHS*. Conference proceedings. London: King's Fund College.

Newson S W B (1982) *Infection Control in Cardiac Surgery. Aspects of Infection Control.* Macclesfield: ICI plc.

Russell A D, Hammond S A and Morgan J R (1986) Bacterial resistance and disinfectants. *Journal of Hospital Infection*, **7**: 213–225.

Sills G A (1986) Sterilisation. *Nursing*, **3**(3): 109–110.

Simmons B (1987) The case for re-use. *Nursing Times*, **83**(11): 26–29.

Simmons B L (1984) The need to reprocess disposable equipment (The Kelsey Lecture). *Journal of Sterile Services Management*, **2**(3): 13–15.

Stuart R C (1979) *The Health and Safety at Work (etc) Act 1974 and its Implications for the NHS.* Paper presented at the Infection Control Nurses Annual Conference 1979.

Street H (1977) *The Need for a Disinfectant Policy.* Paper presented at the Infection Control Nurses Association Annual Conference 1977.

Taylor L J (1979) *Hospital Laundry.* Paper presented at the Infection Control Nurses Association Annual Conference 1979.

Towers A G (1983) *Prevention. A Seminar on the Control of Hospital Acquired Infections.* London: Update Publications.

Walters E M (1980) *The Infection Control Nurse in the UK. Aspects of Infection Control.* Macclesfield: ICI plc.

6

Laboratory Intervention

Microbiological analysis may be requested by the clinician in charge of a patient for a number of reasons. Tests may be carried out to determine which particular organism is causing an obvious infection or to confirm or eliminate a specific site or system as the focus of infection. A test may be prescribed for a patient who has apparently recovered from an infection to check that he is now free of the causative organism.

However, the role of the laboratory is more extensive than just identification of organisms. The microbiologist is available for consultation with clinicians about the suitability of certain tests, for expert interpretation of laboratory findings or for advice on therapy. In the UK, the microbiologist is usually the hospital's infection control officer who will monitor and collate laboratory report information in pursuit of the prevention and control of hospital-acquired infection (see chapter 5).

Most UK hospitals now also have an infection control nurse (ICN) in post. He or she is able to provide a valuable link between the nursing staff and the laboratory. The ICN will use the laboratory results to advise on isolation procedures, wound dressings, sterilisation and disinfection techniques, etc. (Ayliffe et al, 1982). The laboratory findings will, therefore, have a considerable effect on patient care, and laboratory research currently being conducted, for instance, on epidemiology or antibiotic prescribing will affect the future care of patients.

Success in the laboratory is dependent on correct collection and transport of clinical specimens and swabs (Shanson, 1982). Collection of most specimens is usually the responsibility of the nursing staff, and it must be remembered that inadequate specimens will only produce meaningless results. While laboratories have their own local procedures for specimen collection, the basic principles are standard because they are governed by the properties of the particular organism being studied.

The concepts of 'germs' and 'laboratory tests' can be frightening for people who are ill. Reassurance is best achieved by involving the patient in the procedure and by explaining what specimen is required and what will subsequently happen to it.

PRINCIPLES FOR THE COLLECTION OF SPECIMENS

Good quality specimens are obtained when the following principles are adhered to:

● The correct specimen must be taken at the correct time

- The specimen should be uncontaminated by the normal flora of the patient or the person collecting the specimen
- An adequate quantity and appropriate number of specimens need to be sent
- The specimen must be safely contained and clearly labelled

What Type of Specimen?

The correct type of specimen should always be obtained. Contrary to popular belief, it is not true that any specimen is better than no specimen at all, as demonstrated by the large number of useless specimens of saliva rather than sputum that are received in the laboratory. Staff should always consult the laboratory if they are unsure of the type of specimen to collect.

How to Obtain Specimens

People taking specimens have a tendency to overfill containers and this may result in spillage on opening. Although it is generally the rule that the more material sent for examination the greater is the chance of isolating a causative organism, there are limitations to this. If the recommended container is three-quarters full, this will easily be sufficient.

Specimen containers should be securely closed and the outside must not be contaminated. This will avoid the spread of pathogens to porters, laboratory staff and the environment. Every specimen should be clearly identified by a label giving the patient's name and location, the type of specimen, and the date and time of collection.

Contamination of Specimens

Samples are readily contaminated by poor techniques such as in the case of a mid-stream specimen of urine (MSU), allowing urine to flow over the vulva before collection in the appropriate vessel. Specimens should be placed in sterile laboratory containers, with the exception of faeces and sputum which need only clean containers. The technique used must not expose the patient to an increased risk of infection. A survey by Timoney (1987) demonstrated that a high percentage of nurses still obtain specimens from catheterised patients by disconnecting the drainage bag from the catheter. Such a break in the closed drainage system may give bacteria a portal of entry to the patient's bladder, leading to urinary tract infections.

When to Obtain Specimens

Specimens for bacterial culture should be taken before the start of antibiotic therapy. Small doses of antibiotics may damage organisms so that they may not grow in culture media, even though the antibiotic might not necessarily have had any useful clinical effect. When it is necessary to run a test during a course of antibiotics, the specimen should be collected just before an antibiotic dose is given.

Routine specimens should be taken as close as possible to the times of routine transportation. The sooner specimens reach the laboratory, the greater the chance of any organisms present surviving and being identified.

Specimens Awaiting Collection

Unfortunately, many specimens awaiting collection are left on warm specimen shelves which may result in the death of sensitive organisms. Conversely, overgrowth by normal flora may occur, which is often the case with specimens of warm urine which have been left to stand.

With the exception of blood culture samples, which should be placed in an incubator at 37°C, and stools for amoeba, specimens which cannot be sent to the laboratory within a short space of time should be placed in a specimen refrigerator at 4°C to delay growth of bacteria other than the suspected pathogen. Many laboratories issue transport medium for use with swabs, the aim of which is to preserve the organisms in the same condition and numbers as when present in the patient. Swabs in transport medium need not be refrigerated or incubated and should be plated out in the laboratory within 24 hours of being obtained.

All the principles described above should be borne in mind by nurses when obtaining or assisting in the collection of the samples described below.

COLLECTION OF SPECIFIC SPECIMENS

Urine Sampling

A mid-stream specimen of urine (MSU) is the best sample for laboratory examination. Prior to collection the genital area of the patient should be cleaned with soap and water; antiseptics should be avoided as they will interfere with the result. In male patients, the prepuce should be retracted and the glans penis washed. The collection of an uncontaminated MSU from a woman is not easy and nursing supervision should be given whenever possible. The vulva should be cleaned, first the outer labia and then the inner, from front to back to prevent contamination by perineal organisms. The labia should be separated when the specimen is passed to avoid contamination with the patient's skin flora.

The initial part of the urine sample should be discarded and the middle portion of the stream collected directly into a wide-mouthed *sterile* container.

Specimens of urine from a catheterised patient (CSUs) should be obtained by aspiration with a 5ml sterile needle and syringe from the self-sealing sleeve in the drainage tubing. If necessary, the tube should be clamped below the level of the sleeve to allow urine to collect. The sleeve should then be cleaned with alcohol and the hypodermic needle inserted at an angle of 45° through the sample area of the sleeve, taking care not to perforate the far side wall of the tubing. The catheter should never be disconnected to obtain a specimen because this will break the closed system and serve as a portal of entry for organisms. The sample should not be taken from the drainage bag as this will not reflect the bacteria actually present in the bladder (Ayton, 1982).

For culture of tuberculosis-causing bacteria, the first specimen of urine voided on three consecutive mornings should be sent to the laboratory. The organism is more likely to be detected in concentrated or early morning urine. Tubercle bacilli are difficult to detect in urine so three specimens must be examined before a negative result can be given.

Urine specimens should be examined within two hours of collection, or 24 hours if kept refrigerated at 4°C. Bacteria will multiply and other cells such as leucocytes degenerate if the urine is kept at room temperature.

Faeces

Faeces are usually examined for a bacterial or viral cause of diarrhoea, or the presence of ova, cysts or parasites. Specimens of stool for examination should be sent in clean plastic containers; a spoon is usually provided with the container to aid collection. The presence of urine will not affect the result of most microbiological investigations. Rectal swabs are generally unsuitable for detecting enteric bacteria because the organisms have a poor survival rate on swabs and often the intended rectal swab is, in fact, an anal swab.

Three negative stool specimens are usually required to eliminate an infectious cause for diarrhoea. Pathogens are difficult to detect in faeces due to the high numbers of normal flora and they may only be excreted intermittently. Following salmonella gastroenteritis, many clinicians require three negative stool specimens to be obtained, at weekly intervals, to ensure that the patient is not a carrier of the organism. This protocol is particularly important for patients who are food handlers.

Detection of Amoebae

Entamoeba histolytica (the parasite responsible for amoebic dysentery) exists in two characteristic forms:

1. A free-living motile form
2. As non-motile cysts

It is essential that fresh specimens of stool are examined in the laboratory as motile forms are difficult to recognise when dead and the cystic forms degenerate, albeit slowly. Stools should, therefore, be sent for examination as soon as they are passed. Intermittent excretion of cysts can occur and it may be necessary to examine several specimens before amoebae are detected.

Sputum Examination

Sputum is best obtained early in the morning. The help of a physiotherapist may be enlisted to ensure that a true specimen is obtained and that saliva is not collected in error.

In the investigation of pulmonary tuberculosis, three early morning sputum specimens, taken on different days, are required. This is because identification may be difficult as the tubercle bacillus is often only present in low numbers in the sputum, particularly in the early stages of the disease. If sputum cannot be obtained, gastric aspirate should be collected on three successive mornings before any food or liquid is taken. The total aspirate collected should be sent to the laboratory.

Blood Culture

Organisms are likely to be present in the blood stream in their greatest numbers during a rigor when the patient's temperature is at its highest. Although medical staff take blood samples for culture, the nurse can help by informing the doctor when the patient's temperature is rising. Inoculated bottles should be transported to the laboratory for incubation as soon as possible, accompanied by full details of:

● The date and time of specimen collection
● The date of onset of illness
● The patient's temperature at the time of taking the specimen
● Any possible foci of infection, e.g. a septic lesion or urinary tract infection, and the relevant organism(s) likely to be associated with these
● Antibiotic therapy and the time the last dose was given

An aseptic technique is needed for blood culture collection to avoid contamination and inaccurate results.

Serum Antibodies

Antibodies can be detected in serum and their detection can give a useful indication of active infection or immunity. For this investigation, 10 ml of venous blood should be taken, which is evacuated into a dry tube or bottle containing no anticoagulant and allowed to clot.

As specific antibodies do not appear in the serum for several days, it is the usual procedure to take blood at the beginning of an illness and then again after 10 days; the specimens are examined together in the laboratory. An increase in the amount (titre) of antibody in the second specimen will be an indicator of continued stimulation by the organism which must, therefore, still be present in the patient. By comparing two specimens in this way, more information is gained than by examining a single sample which gives no indication as to whether infection is current or old, whether raised antibody levels reflect an earlier illness, or whether a serum sample has been taken too early in the infection to detect antibodies.

It is important that samples are accompanied by full details of:

● The date of onset of the illness
● The clinical history
● Any previous attack of the disease or history of immunisation

The dosage of certain antibiotics, for example, gentamicin, is controlled by the estimation of serum levels of the drug. A certain serum concentration must be attained for the drug to be clinically effective, but too high a level gives rise to toxic side-effects. Samples are taken before a dose of antibiotic is due (**trough** level) and after a dose is given (**peak** level). Trough and peak levels are usually reported in μg/ml ($1 \mu g = 10^{-6}$g). These levels are a guide to the clinician prescribing the drug.

COLLECTION OF SWABS

Samples to be analysed in the laboratory are usually collected using standard swabs.

Collection of Swabs for Bacterial Investigation

All swabs should ideally be placed in a transport medium immediately after collection as this improves the survival rate of organisms during their transport to the laboratory. Stuart's or a similar medium (e.g. Transwab) is suitable for most bacteria.

Nasal Swabs

The normal, healthy nose is virtually dry so, when screening is carried out to check for staphylococcal carriage, the swab should be moistened with sterile distilled water. In this case, nasal swabs should be taken from the anteria nares; the swab is directed upwards in the tip of the nose and gently rotated to collect any secretion present (figure 6.1).

In other circumstances, it is generally important to ensure that the swab reaches as far back as possible on each side. This can usually be done by tilting the patient's head back and gently rotating the swab. With babies and very young children, standard wooden swab sticks are often too large to enter the nostrils and many

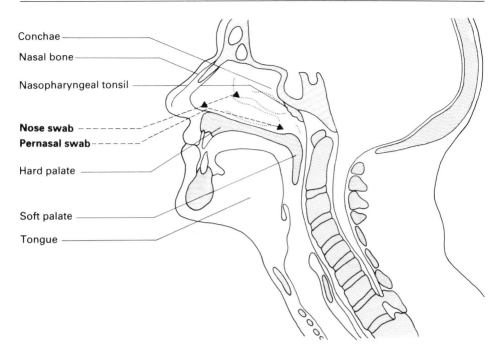

Conchae
Nasal bone
Nasopharyngeal tonsil
Nose swab
Pernasal swab
Hard palate
Soft palate
Tongue

Fig 6.1 Areas to be swabbed when sampling the nose
(From Ayton, 1982. Reproduced by kind permission of *Nursing*)

hospitals supply fine wire swabholders covered with a tiny wisp of cotton wool. Care is needed when using these to avoid damage to the delicate mucous membranes.

Throat Swabs

To obtain a throat swab, the patient is placed facing a strong source of light and the tongue is depressed. Care should be taken to avoid touching the mouth or tongue with the swab which should be gently rubbed over the pillars of the fauces and any area with a lesion or visible exudate.

In practice nasal and throat swabs are usually taken together, one swab for both tonsils and one for both nostrils; organisms causing sore throats are frequently carried in the nose and failure to take nasal swabs may mean that such organisms are missed (figure 6.2).

Pernasal Swabs

A pernasal (cough) swab should be taken in cases of suspected whooping cough, most often in children. A microbiologist or trained laboratory worker usually obtains such specimens. A small swab on a flexible wire is introduced into one nostril and passed into the nasopharynx while an assistant holds the child's head

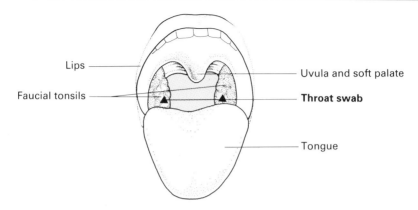

Fig 6.2   Area to be swabbed when sampling the throat
(From Ayton, 1982. Reproduced by kind permission of *Nursing*)

still. The child will inevitably cough; the swab is then withdrawn and placed in charcoal transport medium before being sent to the laboratory.

Eye Swabs

Unsatisfactory results are often obtained with eye swabs due to the action of lysozyme contained in the tears. Conjunctival scrapings are preferred and should be taken using a platinum or plastic loop, then being plated out directly on culture medium. This is usually carried out by medical staff in eye clinics or wards.

Standard swabbing of eye exudate is usually sufficient for the isolation of possible causative organisms (e.g. staphylococci and coliforms) from babies with 'sticky eye'.

Ear Swabs

When otitis externa is thought to be present, a swab of the outer ear should be carefully taken. A deeper swab is required when otitis media is suspected and a speculum should be used to obtain the specimen (figure 6.3).

Vaginal Swabs

A speculum is essential to obtain a high vaginal or cervical swab. Cervical, urethral and vaginal swabs should be broken off in Stuart's transport medium.

Swabs of Pus and Wound Exudate

A wound swab should be obtained before the wound is cleaned and should be taken directly from the infected site, avoiding the undamaged skin and mucous membranes.

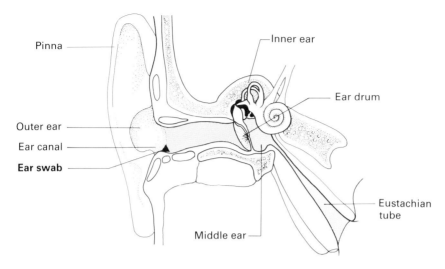

Fig 6.3   Area to be swabbed when sampling the outer ear
(From Ayton, 1982. Reproduced by kind permission of *Nursing*)

Samples of pus or excised tissue are much better for laboratory investigation, particularly for the isolation of anaerobes.

Collection of Specimens for Fungal Investigation

Most specimens can be collected in the same way as those for bacteriological examination as yeasts and fungi will often be detected in routine examination of sputum, swabs, etc. When fungal infections such as ringworm are suspected the specimens should be collected in clean, dry containers. Part of the specimen received will be cultured directly and the other treated with potassium hydroxide and examined under the microscope.

Skin

Skin scrapings should be taken from the active periphery of skin lesions with a blunt scalpel.

Hair

Hairs which show signs of such infection or abnormality should be removed with forceps for examination. Most infections will be of the scalp, so it is important to remove the hair at the root so this can be examined.

Nails

Full thickness clippings or thick shavings are taken from affected nails.

Collection of Specimens for Viral Investigation

Specialist virus laboratories should be consulted before specimens are taken. Specimens should be delivered to the laboratory within one hour of collection, or refrigerated at 4°C if there is to be a delay. The virologist will need to know the date of onset of illness and the patient's immunisation record, particularly any inoculation within the previous month. Due to the specialist nature of the laboratory specimens, staff often prefer to visit the ward to obtain the specimen themselves. If viral disease is thought to be present, several different specimens may need to be taken as the site of infection may not always be apparent.

When investigating a viral infection, culture is only one of a number of laboratory tests that may be employed (table 6.1).

THE LABORATORY REQUEST FORM

Requests for laboratory investigations are made by the medical staff. When a specimen is obtained by the nursing staff, the nurse must enter details of the date and time of collection of the specimen on the laboratory request form. Accurate information will help laboratory staff to select the most appropriate tests and

Table 6.1   Investigations for viral infections

Infections	Specimen	Test	Viruses
Respiratory tract infection	Throat swab, nasopharyngeal washings	Culture	Influenza, para-influenza, adeno- and rhino-respiratory synctial viruses, some enteroviruses
Respiratory tract infection	Paired sera	Serology	Influenza, para-influenza, adenovirus, respiratory synctial viruses, mumps
Vesicular skin lesion	Vesicular fluid/ scrapings	Electron microscopy	Herpes simplex virus, varicella zoster virus
	Paired sera	Culture	Herpes simplex virus, varicella zoster virus
		Serology	Herpes simplex virus, varicella zoster virus
Erythematous skin rash	Paired sera	Serology	Measles, rubella
Congenital infections	Throat swab, urine	Culture	Cytomegalovirus, rubella
	Paired sera of mother and baby	Serology	Cytomegalovirus, rubella
Hepatitis	Serum	Serology	Hepatitis B antigen/antibody, hepatitis A antibody
Eye infections	Conjunctival scrapings	Culture	Herpes simplex virus, adenovirus
Gastroenteritis	Faeces	Electron microscopy	Rotavirus, calicivirus, astrovirus, coronavirus, small round virus

(From Ayton, 1982. Reproduced by kind permission of *Nursing*)

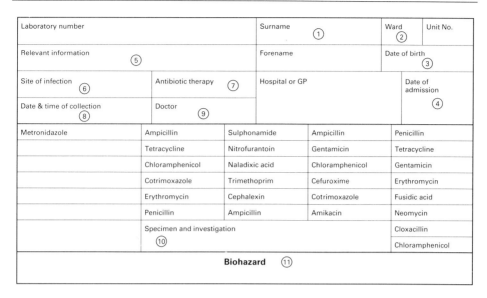

Fig 6.4   Sample laboratory request form

investigations and to interpret results. The standard request form (figure 6.4) is designed for this purpose. It is important that the following information is included:

1. *The patient's name and hospital number*   This may seem obvious but it is surprising how often this important detail is omitted. The hospital number may be used for filing purposes or to distinguish between people of the same name.

2. *Ward name or number*   This allows the report to be returned to the ward with minimum delay.

3. *Patient's date of birth*   The laboratory will investigate for different pathogens in accordance with the patient's age; for instance, examination of stools for enteropathogenic *E. coli* would only be relevant in infants.

4. *Date of admission to hospital*   This is helpful to infection control staff in their surveillance of hospital-acquired infections.

5. *Relevant information*   The key word here is 'relevant'. This section is often blank or full of very interesting information about the patient which is totally unrelated to the specimen. For example wound swab 'relevant' information would not include diarrhoea and vomiting information. The information given in this section will affect how the specimen is processed.

6. *Site of infection*   This information should be as specific as possible to help laboratory staff in distinguishing pathogens from normal flora. *Staph. aureus* may be considered normal flora in the nose but would be reported as a possible pathogen in a leg ulcer. If several wounds are present, it should be stated which swab comes from which site.

7. *Antibiotic therapy*   Laboratory results can be misleading unless the antibiotic therapy which the patient is receiving is stated. Even small doses of antibiotics can inhibit the growth of disease-causing organisms in a laboratory setting. Strains may be selected out in the laboratory which are not the cause of the problem, e.g. ampicillin-resistant *Klebsiella* species are common in the sputum of patients treated with ampicillin but are rarely a cause of chest infection.

8. *Date and time of collection of the specimen*   This is important as different organisms survive for varying periods and overgrowth of a contaminant can often occur which will affect the interpretation made by laboratory staff.

9. *The doctor requesting the investigation*   This enables laboratory staff to obtain further information or communicate important results quickly to the doctor concerned.

10. *Specimen type and investigation requested*   The form should state clearly what the specimen is and where it has been taken from as most swabs look the same in the laboratory. It must be made clear whether the specimen is for microculture and antibiotic sensitivity testing (MC and S), for virology or for serology.

11. *Biohazard specimens*   Forms accompanying biohazard specimens, such as blood from a hepatitis B-infected patient or HIV antibody positive patient, or stool from a known salmonella excreter, should be clearly labelled with a hazard notice in addition to labelling the specimen itself. Most hospitals have special adhesive labels for this purpose. All biohazard specimens should be sent to the laboratory in dual-compartment, plastic specimen bags. This system provides protection for portering staff from any accidental spillage and prevents contamination of the accompanying request form. Many hospitals now use dual-compartment bags for transport of all specimens.

TRANSPORT OF SPECIMENS TO THE LABORATORY

Any potentally infectious material that is being transported from place to place could present a hazard to the health of people who are in contact with it. Packaging and transport of specimens therefore needs to be strictly regulated. The (Howie) Code of Practice (Department of Health and Social Security, 1978) specifies the precautions to be taken in the UK when transporting specimens. Porters or other staff who carry specimens should wear overalls. They should be warned about the possible hazards of the specimens they are carrying and instructed in frequent hand-washing. Specimens should never be taken into canteens or through kitchens.

Specimen containers should be robust and leak-proof. Screw-capped plastic containers are now quite extensively used, and they come in a wide range of shapes and sizes (figure 6.5). Although they are generally robust, care should be taken to screw the cap on fully to avoid leakage. Specimen containers should not be overfilled. This is particularly important with stool specimens as fermentation with

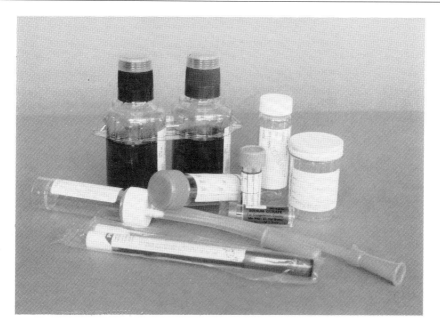

Fig 6.5   Screwcapped containers

considerable gas production may occur during transit and the pressure may cause leakage or even force the cap off the bottle or tube.

The DHSS Code of Practice also insists that leak-proof trays or boxes should be provided for the transport of specimens from wards to the laboratory. Containers need to be both washable and autoclavable so that routine cleaning and spillages can be easily dealt with. Specimens should be placed upright in these containers; alternatively, dual-compartment plastic bags can be used. This will protect anyone who handles the specimen during its journey to the laboratory but, to protect laboratory staff who handle the specimen, care should still be taken to avoid contamination of the outside of the container.

Specimens should be obtained as close to the time of the hospital's collection round as possible. This will help to ensure that they are transported by staff who are aware of necessary precautions and of the need for good quality specimens to be received by the laboratory. When an emergency examination of a specimen is required outside laboratory opening hours, an on-call service is available. Other specimens that do not require immediate examination, e.g. urine or sputum taken before antibiotic therapy is commenced, should be stored in a designated ward or laboratory fridge. Blood culture specimens taken outside hours should be stored in laboratory incubators. Where ward staff are transporting such specimens to the laboratory the precautions outlined previously will naturally still apply.

Transport Between Hospitals

Pathological specimens are frequently conveyed from one hospital to another because of the centralisation of laboratory services. The usual means of transport is by hospital van or car. Specimens should be packed in metal or plastic boxes with fastening lids which should be clearly marked with the name and address of the laboratory to which they are travelling.

Postal Transportation

Specimens may need to be sent to a hospital laboratory by general practitioners, or by a hospital laboratory to a reference laboratory. Clear guidelines are given by the Post Office as to what specimens may be sent and the method of packaging. In principle the container must be robust and securely closed. It must be cocooned in enough absorbent packing material to retain the contents should they leak or the container be broken.

LABORATORY INVESTIGATIONS

The laboratory methods used to identify disease-causing microorganisms in specimens can be considered in seven categories:

1. Macroscopy
2. Microscopy
3. Culture
4. Biochemical tests
5. Resistance
6. Serology
7. Pathogenicity tests in experimental animals

Macroscopy

Direct examination of a specimen can give immediate clues to the presence of an infection. Purulent sputum or turbid cerebrospinal fluid (CSF) is immediate evidence of infection. A foul-smelling sample of pus may indicate anaerobic organisms. Blood and mucus in a liquid stool specimen would suggest dysentery. Occasionally, a diagnosis can even be made with the naked eye if, for example, a tapeworm segment or roundworm is apparent in a specimen of faeces. Most specimens will, however, need to be examined under a microscope.

Microscopy

Some specimens may be examined directly (**unstained**) but, for clear identification, most specimens require the addition of a dye (**stain**).

Unstained (Wet) Films

Drops of a liquid specimen are placed on a glass slide which is covered with a coverslip and examined with the high-power dry objective ($\times 40$) of the microscope. A ten-fold multiplying ($\times 10$) eye-piece is then used to give a final 400-fold magnification. By this method, it is possible to determine the size and shape of the organisms and whether or not they are motile. This technique is used in the examination of:

- CSF, urine or body fluids when looking for pus cells and organisms
- Faeces when investigating for ova or cysts
- Vaginal secretions to look for trichomonas and candida
- Skin, nails and hair (after cleaning in warm potassium hydroxide) if fungal infection is suspected

Stained (Dry) Films

Bacteria are commonly examined by fixing them to a glass slide (usually by heat) and applying stains. A higher magnification can be obtained than for wet films as dry films can be examined under oil. The oil immersion objective ($\times 100$) of the microscope is used with a bright light source. If a $\times 10$ eye-piece is added to this, a final magnification of $\times 1000$ can be achieved.

The most commonly used stain is **Gram's stain** (see chapter 2). This determines the predominant types of bacterial pathogen (**Gram-positive** or **Gram-negative**) present in pus, sputum, CSF or specimens from other sites. Gram-staining can be of life-saving importance, for example, in the rapid diagnosis of bacterial meningitis in a child by examining his CSF.

The tubercle bacillus (*Mycobacterium tuberculosis*) and related organisms are stained only with difficulty by Gram's stain. They can, however, be reliably stained by hot, strong carbol fuchsin. This dye cannot be removed by acid and alcohol. This is the basis of the **Ziehl–Nielsen** stain for tubercle organisms. In the laboratory report, the results of this examination are often abbreviated to ZN positive (Ziehl–Nielsen positive) or AFB positive (acid-fast bacillus positive). A fluorescent stain (auramine phenol) is now also commonly used.

A number of other specialised stains, such as the Giemsa stain used to detect malarial parasites in the blood, are also available in the laboratory. With many parasitic infections, staining is the only method of laboratory diagnosis as the organisms cannot be cultured and serology is not always helpful.

Dark Ground Microscopy

This technique, in which bacteria appear brightly illuminated against a dark background, is used to visualise organisms that cannot readily be seen by a light microscope. It is mainly used to look for the spirochaete *Treponema pallidum* in suspected primary or secondary syphilitic lesions.

Immunofluorescence Microscopy

This is useful for the rapid diagnosis of a number of viral infections. The technique employs antibody labelled with fluorescent dye to detect specific antigens and so identify organisms. It aids in the detection of respiratory syncytial virus, herpes simplex, rabies virus in brain biopsy specimens and chlamydia in conjunctival scrapings.

Electron Microscopy

In this method, a beam of electrons is used rather than a ray of light. The beam passes through a series of electromagnetic fields which focus it onto the specimen. After it has passed through the material to be examined, the beam produces a visible image on a fluorescent screen or gives rise to photographs that can be enlarged. Magnification levels of 300 000 times or more (compared with 1500-fold for a light microscope) can be achieved.

Electron microscopy is commonly used in the laboratory for the rapid diagnosis of rotavirus or herpes infections because of the distinctive morphology of these viruses.

Culture

Both bacteria and viruses can be cultured to give additional information about the pathogen present.

Bacterial Culture

Bacteria can be distinguished by the manner in which they grow in the laboratory. In order to determine these cultural characteristics, infected material is introduced into a suitable liquid or solid medium. The medium is basically a nutrient broth solidified, if necessary, by the addition of a gelatin-like substance called **agar**. The nutrient broth provides protein, carbohydrate and other factors at a pH suitable for bacterial growth. Most bacteria isolated from humans either require blood for their growth or show an improved growth on blood-containing media (**blood agar**).

Other types of medium are also available. MacConkey medium (bile-salt lactose agar) promotes the growth of intestinal organisms. Some media are selective for growth of a particular organism in preference to others. Deoxycholate-citrate agar, for example, is used for selectively growing salmonella or shigella in preference to the normal bowel flora. Fluid media are useful when bacteria are present only in small numbers. If the medium is adapted with special constituents (e.g. sugars), it can also be employed to determine the biochemical activities of the bacteria.

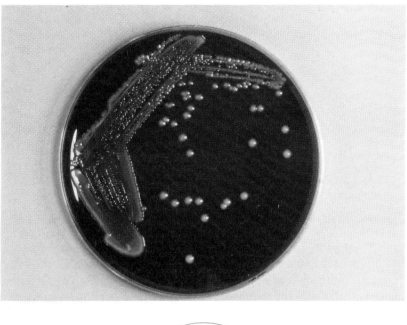

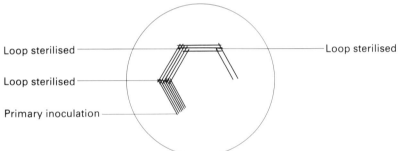

Loop sterilised ——————————————————— Loop sterilised

Loop sterilised ——————

Primary inoculation ——————

Fig 6.6   Diagram illustrating the method used to obtain separate bacterial colonies on a solid medium
using a wire loop

Growth on solid media is predominantly used in the initial stage of identification.
The sample of infected material is cultured on a plate (**petri dish**) containing the
culture medium. The specimen is **plated out** or stroked onto the medium with a
sterilised wire loop in such a way that the initial inoculum is reduced in successive
stages (figure 6.6). The plates are then incubated at 37°C for 18 to 24 hours. Where
anaerobic organisms, e.g. *Clostridium tetani*, are expected, the plates are incubated
in an atmosphere where the oxygen has been replaced with other gases. This is
usually a special cabinet fed with a mixture of hydrogen, nitrogen and carbon
dioxide.

Some organisms grow slowly and often no growth is visible to the naked eye even
after 24 hours. With other organisms, there will be heaped colonies of growing
organisms, ranging from 0.1 to 4 mm in diameter, along the lines of inoculation.

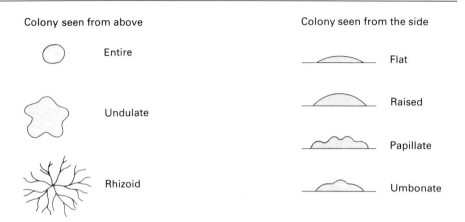

Fig 6.7   Differentiation of bacteria by shape of the colonies observed on solid media

These colonies, each containing many organisms all of one kind, have developed by division of the initial bacteria put on with the loop. Their size, shape, colour, consistency and effect on the surrounding medium are all of importance and can be used to characterise the species (figure 6.7).

Unless a selective medium has been used, the culture will be a mixture of colonies of different bacteria, including the normal flora. A pure culture can be obtained by placing isolated bacterial colonies on a fresh solid medium; this stage is necessary for full bacterial identification.

Viral Culture

Unlike bacteria, viruses cannot be grown on artificial cell-free media. They are cultured using one of the following techniques:

- Tissue culture
- Chick embryo culture
- Inoculation of laboratory animals

These are all somewhat complex techniques and will not be considered further here (for a detailed explanation see Timbury, 1980).

Biochemical Tests

Biochemical tests are useful in differentiating one organism from another, particularly the Gram-negative bacilli. Most tests are designed to detect the presence of enzymes which bring about a specific chemical reaction. They are devised so that a visible change occurs, e.g. pH change or gas production.

In this way, species of the shigella group of organisms, for example, can be differentiated by their carbohydrate metabolism. Only *Shigella sonnei* and *Shigella flexneri* are able to ferment the sugar mannitol, and can therefore be distinguished from other shigellae if grown on a mannitol-containing medium. The fermentation can be identified if an indicator is added that will demonstrate acid production by its change in colour.

There are many other examples of such diagnostic tests, and most laboratories now use commercially prepared kits which enable a range of tests to be carried out rapidly and accurately.

Resistance

The resistance of an organism to temperature, drying, acid, antiseptics, dyes, chemotherapeutic agents and antibiotics can be a useful diagnostic tool.

Although the sensitivity of various organisms to antibiotics may be of value in differentiating strains, it is of more importance as a guide to therapy.

The most widely used method to test antibiotic sensitivity is **disc diffusion** (see chapter 7 for a more detailed description). The petri dish is completely inoculated with the test organism and paper discs impregnated with antibiotic solutions (at concentrations related to blood or urine levels) are placed on the surface of the medium. An inhibition of growth around the disc (shown by a clear zone) indicates that the organism is sensitive to the antibiotic (figure 6.8).

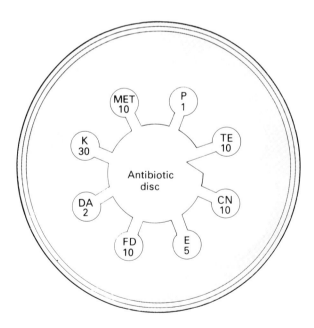

Fig 6.8   Antibiotic sensitivity tests. Antibiotic-impregnated discs are placed on a lawn of the test organism. Resistance is shown by growth of the organism right up to the disc

Serology

An organism isolated from infected material contains numerous antigens. These can be mixed with serum containing known specific antibodies, prepared by the injection of a known organism into an experimental animal and then collection of its serum. If the unknown organism reacts with the specific antiserum, the antigens in the unknown organism must be the same as, or closely related to, those which were used to immunise the experimental animal.

Antigen–antibody reactions are used a great deal in bacteriology. The union of antigen with antibody is associated with an altered physical state of the mixture such as a clumping of red blood cells. This principle forms the basis of the **anti-streptolysin O** (ASO) titre test used when possible indirect complications of *Streptococcus pyogenes* infection, such as rheumatic fever or acute glomerulonephritis, are suspected. (Streptolysin O is a toxin produced by streptococci which destroys red blood cells.)

Pathogenicity Tests in Experimental Animals

In the UK, improvements in laboratory techniques mean that experimental animals are now rarely used to identify pathogens. However, there are a few infectious agents that can only be detected by their production of the disease in an experimental animal which is known to be susceptible. Tissues from the animal may show changes typical of the disease. For example, when tubercle bacilli cannot be found in the urine, tuberculosis may sometimes be identified by injecting some of the infected fluid into a guinea-pig which will develop the illness.

Bacterial Typing

When it is necessary for epidemiological reasons to identify individual stains – or types – of bacteria within a species, the following methods can be used:

1. *Antigenic typing* This involves the identification of the antigens which distinguish different strains of bacteria.

2. *Bacteriophage typing* Bacterial strains are identified by their varying susceptibilities to a series of bacterial viruses or bacteriophages, as shown by differing patterns of bacterial lysis using more than one phage.

3. *Bacteriocine typing* Strains are identified by the release of bacteriocines which inhibit the growth of other members of the same species, but not of the same strain.

The bacteriologist employs some or all of the above laboratory methods to investigate organisms present in the material which is sent to him, but their identification may take some time. Occasionally, organisms can be seen in direct films of the material and their appearance will be diagnostic. More commonly, 18 hours are necessary for the organism to be grown on media and only then can the various differential tests be applied and the resulting report returned to the ward or department.

THE LABORATORY REPORT

While nurses need to know how to obtain specimens and what happens to them in the laboratory, it is essential that they are also able to interpret laboratory reports and incorporate the information into nursing care plans. Does the report indicate that the patient has an infection? Will it be a potential source of cross-infection to others? What modification should be made to the care plan? A problem-solving approach to nursing requires an understanding of the information received, especially with regard to infection risk factors.

Information Contained in the Report

Macroscopy

The laboratory may comment on the gross appearance of the specimen. This will help the clinician to assess the significance of the report; for example, *Staphylococcus aureus* reported in saliva may not be significant but in sputum it is a likely cause of severe chest infection.

Microscopy

The laboratory will report on the presence of cells, casts or crystals, yeasts or fungi, and parasites or their ova observed on prepared slides viewed under the microscope. This will also help in the clinical interpretation of the report, e.g. in the case of a wound swab, pus cells recorded from the site would indicate infection rather than colonisation.

Culture

After culturing, the organism can be identified and named, e.g. as streptococcus (the family name). This may be followed by the abbreviation of sp. which means species (singular; spp. = species, plural), or the organism may be further identified as a member of a particular species or family, e.g. *Strep. faecalis* or *Strep. pyogenes*.

The growth of the organism may be described qualitatively as heavy (+++), moderate (++), or low (+). It may also be described numerically; for example, the number of bacteria per ml of urine may be expressed as $>10^5$/ml (i.e. more than 100 000 organisms in 1 ml of urine). This would be considered as a significant number of bacteria in urine and may indicate a urinary tract infection.

The laboratory may report on the presence or absence of a particular organism (in a screening test) if requested by the clinician. For example the report may state 'No salmonella spp. isolated'.

Antibiotic Sensitivity

The sensitivity of a pathogen to a range of antibiotics is reported in an abbreviated form on the report as:

- S = sensitive
- R = resistant

This serves as a guide to the clinician who will prescribe if necessary.

Interpretation of Laboratory Reports

Laboratory reports serve several functions. They may:

- Be diagnostic or contribute towards establishing a diagnosis
- Specify suitable antibiotic prescribing
- Determine the medical or nursing management of the patient
- Be used in series as a measure of the patient's progress

The clinical condition of the patient must always be considered when interpreting laboratory reports. When interpretation is not straightforward, the advice of the microbiologist should be sought. *Staph. aureus* reported in a septic wound may be the obvious causal pathogen, but is the *N. meningitidis* from the throat of a patient with meningitis the pathogen or normal flora? Ampicillin-resistant klebsiella species isolated from a sputum specimen of a patient on ampicillin therapy may not be the organism causing an infection, but may rather result from overgrowth of normal flora in a poor specimen.

Laboratory number Form 1			Surname SMITH		Ward D20	Unit No. 551260
Relevant information Laparotomy 17.3.87			Forename Jane		Consultant Mr. Jones	
Site of infection Abdominal wound	Antibiotic therapy None		Hospital or GP D.R.H.		Date of birth 15.01.50	
Date & time of collection 24.3.87 09.30 hours	Doctor Dr James				Date of admission 16.3.87	
Micro: + + + pus cells Culture: *Staph. aureus*						
Metronidazole	Ampicillin	Sulphonamide	Ampicillin		Penicillin	R
	Tetracycline	Nitrofurantoin	Gentamicin		Tetracycline	S
	Chloramphenicol	Naladixic acid	Chloramphenicol		Gentamicin	S
	Cotrimoxazole	Trimethoprim	Cefuroxime		Erythromycin	S
	Erythromycin	Cephalexin	Cotrimoxazole		Fusidic acid	S
	Penicillin	Ampicillin	Amikacin		Neomycin	S
	Specimen and investigation Wound swab for MC + S please				Cloxacillin	S
					Chloramphenicol	S

Fig 6.9   Example 1

Laboratory number
    Form 2
		Surname
		    KAUR
			Ward
			    D21
				Unit No.
				    562320

Relevant information
    Ulcer (R) leg
		Forename
		    Kulwinder
			Consultant
			    Dr Jones	

Site of infection
    ? ulcer
	Antibiotic therapy
	    None
		Hospital or GP
		
		    D.R.H.
			Date of birth
			    20.3.35	

Date & time of collection
    12.3.87   10.00 a.m.
	Doctor
	    Dr James
			Date of admission
			    1.3.87	

Micro: No pus cells Culture: ± *Staph. aureus*					
Metronidazole	Ampicillin	Sulphonamide	Ampicillin	Penicillin	R
	Tetracycline	Nitrofurantoin	Gentamicin	Tetracycline	S
	Chloramphenicol	Naladixic acid	Chloramphenicol	Gentamicin	S
	Cotrimoxazole	Trimethoprim	Cefuroxime	Erythromycin	S
	Erythromycin	Cephalexin	Cotrimoxazole	Fusidic acid	S
	Penicillin	Ampicillin	Amikacin	Neomycin	S
	Specimen and investigation Wound swab for MC + S please			Cloxacillin	S
				Chloramphenicol	S

Fig 6.10   Example 2

The fact that a pathogen and antibiotic sensitivities are indicated on the report does not necessarily imply that the patient must be given therapy. He may already be recovering from the infection or may only have been colonised by the organism. The fact that no organism was isolated does not necessarily mean that the site was sterile; this could be the result of poor technique in obtaining the specimen.

Figures 6.9 to 6.12 are given as an exercise in interpreting laboratory reports. How would these reports affect patient care and management?

Laboratory number
    Form 3
		Surname
		    BROWN
			Ward
			    D30
				Unit No.
				    543620

Relevant information
    Drainage of abdominal abscess 12.1.87
    Discharge from wound
		Forename
		    John
			Consultant
			    Dr. Singh	

Site of infection
    Abdominal wound
	Antibiotic therapy
	    None
		Hospital or GP
		
		    D.R.H.
			Date of birth
			    19.3.35	

Date & time of collection
    20.1.87   6.00 am.
	Doctor
	    Dr. James
			Date of admission
			    12.1.87	

Micro: No pus cells. Debris only. Culture : No growth				
Metronidazole	Ampicillin	Sulphonamide	Ampicillin	Penicillin
	Tetracycline	Nitrofurantoin	Gentamicin	Tetracycline
	Chloramphenicol	Naladixic acid	Chloramphenicol	Gentamicin
	Cotrimoxazole	Trimethoprim	Cefuroxime	Erythromycin
	Erythromycin	Cephalexin	Cotrimoxazole	Fusidic acid
	Penicillin	Ampicillin	Amikacin	Neomycin
	Specimen and investigation Pus MC + S please			Cloxacillin
				Chloramphenicol

Fig 6.11   Example 3

Laboratory number Form 4		Surname WHITE		Ward D21	Unit No. 222222
Relevant information Diarrhoea		Forename Mary		Consultant Dr. Singh	
Site of infection ? bowel	Antibiotic therapy None	Hospital or GP D.R.H.		Date of birth 10.5.30	
Date & time of collection 20.3.87 10.00 am.	Doctor Dr James			Date of admission 1.3.87	

Salmonella typhimurium isolated

Metronidazole	Ampicillin	Sulphonamide	Ampicillin		Penicillin
	Tetracycline	Nitrofurantoin	Gentamicin	S	Tetracycline
	Chloramphenicol	Naladixic acid	Chloramphenicol	S	Gentamicin
	Cotrimoxazole	Trimethoprim	Cefuroxime	S	Erythromycin
	Erythromycin	Cephalexin	Cotrimoxazole	S	Fusidic acid
	Penicillin	Ampicillin	Amikacin	S	Neomycin
	Specimen and investigation				Cloxacillin
					Chloramphenicol

Fig 6.12   Example 4

Example 1   The presence of pus cells noted on the report confirms that this is a wound infection, and *Staph. aureus* is the likely pathogen. Antibiotic sensitivities are recorded as it is likely that therapy would be instigated by the clinician. This is not a multi-resistant *Staph. aureus* and, although isolation would not be necessary, particular care would be required to prevent cross-infection, especially during dressing changes. The wound should be assessed regularly and local treatment modified when necessary.

Example 2   *Staph. aureus* is again isolated but it is not clear without a clinical assessment whether this is infecting or only colonising the ulcer. However, the ulcer will need to be closely monitored.

Example 3   No growth at all is recorded from this abdominal wound swab, which could be due to a poorly taken swab. No pus cells are noted but the report of debris indicates that the swab has dried out. Note the early time of collection. This swab may well need to be repeated.

Example 4   This patient will require isolation and precautions against enteric infections to prevent cross-infection. Note the difference between the date of admission and the date the specimen was sent. It is unclear from the form when the patient developed symptoms. Is this a hospital-acquired infection? If the patient was on a general ward, other patients who had been in contact with him will need to be closely observed. Further specimens will be required and the environmental health services must be notified by the clinician.

References

Ayliffe G A J, Collins B J and Taylor L J (1982) *Hospital Acquired Infection: Principles and Prevention*. Bristol: John Wright.

Ayton M (1982) Microbiological investigations. *Nursing*, **2**(8): 226–230.
Department of Health and Social Security (1978) *Code of Practice for Prevention of Infection in Clinical Laboratories and Post-Mortem Rooms* (The Howie Report). London: HMSO.
Shanson D C (1982) *Microbiology in Clinical Practice*. Bristol: John Wright.
Timbury M S (1980) *Notes on Medical Virology*, 6th edn. Edinburgh: Churchill Livingstone.
Timoney R (1987) Looking into the community. *Nursing Times*, **83**(9), *Journal of Infection Control*, pp. 64–71.

Further Reading

Douglas-Sleigh J and Timbury M C (1981) *Notes on Medical Bacteriology*. London: Churchill Livingstone.
Ross P W (1979) *Clinical Bacteriology*. Edinburgh: Churchill Livingstone.
Thomas C G A (1979) *Medical Microbiology*, 4th edn. London: Baillière Tindall.

7

Pharmacological Intervention

Treatment of human infectious diseases has been carried out for as long as civilisation itself, until very recently with uniformly poor results. Over the centuries, there were never-ending attempts to find a substance that would kill invading organisms within the body without damaging the body in the process. Even after the discovery and acceptance of the 'infective organism' theories of disease propounded by Pasteur and Lister in the 1860s, the success of powerfully active substances was marred by their often fatal human toxicity. One example of this was with the use of mercury preparations against syphilitic disease; the syphilis was often cured but usually at the expense of poisoning the patient.

To quote a century-old therapeutic textbook:

● 'Mercury is one of the most valuable drugs we have. It is a direct antidote to the syphilitic virus, it can completely cure the patient, its use must be continued over a long time, but it should never be pushed to salivation.' (Hale White, 1892)

The textbook then goes on to describe the toxicity of such long-term treatment:

● 'The teeth are now loose, the saliva, which is thick and viscid, pours over the mouth . . . these symptoms ended in the falling out of teeth, extensive ulceration of the mouth and tongue, necrosis of the jaw, great weakness, emaciation, anaemia, a watery state of the blood, a liability to haemorrhages, exhaustion and death.'

At the start of the twentieth century, the combination of the developing chemical industry and enquiring scientific minds led to the synthesis and then testing of many completely novel chemical substances. The chemist could now produce derivatives of active but poisonous substances. These preparations were still effective against infective organisms without being toxic to the patient. A safer treatment for syphilis was still being sought and, in 1910, the German chemist Paul Ehrlich produced 605 such derivatives of arsenic before discovering arsphenamine. This compound became known as '606' and was, for many years, to be the main treatment for syphilitic diseases.

The search for such laboratory synthesised antibacterial substances continued, often guided by inspiration. For example, it was realised that dyestuffs for the clothing industry were 'permanent' because they actually bonded to the protein in wool. Perhaps a similar chemical could bind to, and destroy, bacterial protein. In

1935, the red dye sulphamidochrysoidin (Prontosil) was found to be active against infections induced in mice. The active component of this dye was found to be sulphanilamide which, following its use against infections in humans, led to a dramatic decrease in mortality rate.

The impact made by sulphanilamide and the antibacterial agents that followed it is demonstrated most spectacularly by the UK statistics for deaths in children due to infectious disease. In 1940, just as the first antibacterials were becoming available, the death rate was 3000 per million children. By 1970, after a generation had been treated with safe and effective antibacterials, the death rate had dropped eight-fold to 450 per million. Sulphanilamide is reputed to have saved the life of Sir Winston Churchill who, in 1942, was gravely ill with pneumonia.

The first scientific examination and development of a naturally occurring antibacterial substance is attributed to Sir Alexander Fleming with his study of the mould *Penicillium notatum* in the late 1920s. It is interesting to note that folk remedies through the ages have used moulds to treat infected wounds. In the late nineteenth century, the inhibitory effect of mould on bacteria was being examined at laboratory level in several European centres involved in investigation of possible modes of activity. Accounts of Fleming's observations at St Mary's Hospital, London, of the suppression of growth of *Staphylococcus aureus* by a secretion of the penicillium mould are many and certainly varied (figures 7.1 and 7.2). None the less, the coincident timing of Fleming's papers with the developments of pharmaceutical technology led to the production of the first pure, naturally produced antibiotic for clinical use. The term **antibiotic** refers specifically to a naturally occurring substance produced by one type of microorganism that is capable of inhibiting the growth of another type of microorganism.

ON THE ANTIBACTERIAL ACTION OF CULTURES OF A PENICILLIUM, WITH SPECIAL REFERENCE TO THEIR USE IN THE ISOLATION OF *B. INFLUENZÆ.*

ALEXANDER FLEMING, F.R.C.S.

From the Laboratories of the Inoculation Department, St Mary's Hospital, London.

Received for publication May 10th, 1929.

WHILE working with staphylococcus variants a number of culture-plates were set aside on the laboratory bench and examined from time to time. In the examinations these plates were necessarily exposed to the air and they became contaminated with various micro-organisms. It was noticed that around a large colony of a contaminating mould the staphylococcus colonies became transparent and were obviously undergoing lysis (see Fig. 1).

Subcultures of this mould were made and experiments conducted with a view to ascertaining something of the properties of the bacteriolytic substance which had evidently been formed in the mould culture and which had diffused into the surrounding medium. It was found that broth in which the mould had been grown at room temperature for one or two weeks had acquired marked inhibitory, bactericidal and bacteriolytic properties to many of the more common pathogenic bacteria.

Fig 7.1   Title and opening section of Fleming's celebrated paper in the June 1929 issue of *The British Journal of Experimental Pathology*
(From Selwyn, 1980. Reproduced by kind permission of Hodder and Stoughton)

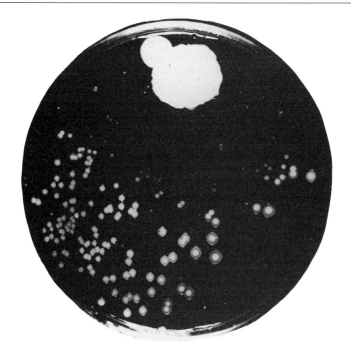

British Journal of Experimental Pathology, Vol. X. No. 3.

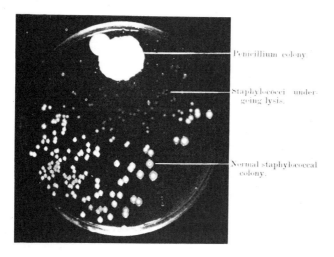

Fig 7.2   Photograph of the original culture of *Staphylococcus aureus* contaminated with
Penicillium notatum
(From Selwyn, 1980. Reproduced by kind permission of Hodder and Stoughton)

There is no doubt that had not the Second World War, with its consequent injury and disease, supplied the greatest possible pressure to obtain antibacterial products, the development of penicillins, including their purification and isolation, might never have taken place. Co-operation between biological scientists and technologists at an international level at that time led to the establishment of the modern, research-based pharmaceutical industry.

Following the discovery, isolation, preparation and successful clinical use of penicillin, the search for more naturally occurring antibiotics began. Extensive investigations were made world-wide, examining microorganisms found in soil samples or even sewage effluent. From soil-borne bacteria came streptomycin, chloramphenicol and tetracycline in the late 1940s, erythromycin and rifampicin in the late 1950s and gentamicin and sodium fusidate in the late 1960s. The cephalosporins were to follow in the 1970s, having been first isolated from a mould growing in the sea near a sewage outfall in Sardinia in 1948.

Each new antibiotic was heralded as being of broader spectrum and inducing lower resistance than its predecessors. Unfortunately, none has fully lived up to its claim, mainly due to the development of bacterial resistance. Penicillin-resistant *Staphylococcus aureus* became a serious problem in hospitals throughout the world in the 1950s. This was soon followed by certain strains of colonic bacteria becoming resistant to several antibiotics simultaneously. Now, in the 1980s, penicillin-resistant organisms are again becoming routinely encountered.

THE RATIONAL USE OF ANTIBACTERIALS

To ensure the safe and effective use of antibacterials it is important to understand many factors, ranging from the mode of action of the drug to the acquiring by the target bacteria of resistance to that drug. The more scientific aspects will be discussed first, before moving on to the application of these principles to clinical situations.

Mode of Action of Antibacterials

Antibacterial agents have widely differing molecular structures (figure 7.3). Such differences make it difficult to assign a simple mode of action, but they do explain differential activity whereby certain antibacterials affect only certain bacteria.

This differential activity may be determined by the barrier presented by the cell wall. A bacterial cell wall is composed of layers of protein complexes, cross-linked to make a large molecule (see chapter 2). The actual structure of these proteins varies between species to the extent that one antibacterial may pass through the cell wall where another may not. The difference in the cell walls is used in broad typing of bacteria with chemical stains. Gram's staining procedure divides bacterial species into two broad groups, depending on whether the stain is retained (Gram-positive) or not retained (Gram-negative) by the cell wall (see chapter 6).

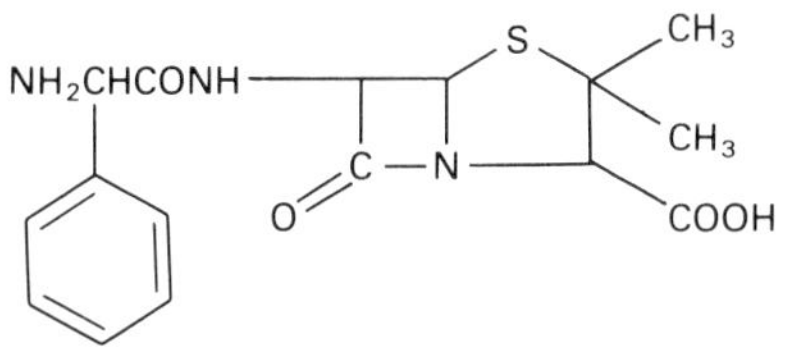

Ampicillin

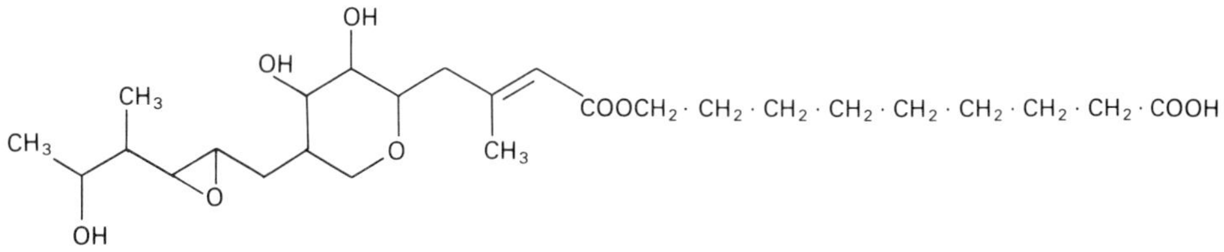

Pseudomonic acid A

Fig 7.3   Structures of ampicillin and pseudomonic acid A

Antibiotic activity can then be related to Gram-staining ability; e.g. erythromycin penetrates the cell wall of Gram-positive bacteria, and is therefore an effective treatment for such infections, but it does not penetrate the cell wall of coliform bacteria so cannot be used for these Gram-negative infections.

Antibacterial activity is conveniently divided into two categories:

- **Bactericidal**, e.g., penicillins, in which the developing cells are actively destroyed
- **Bacteriostatic**, e.g. erythromycin, where cells are not killed but are prevented from replicating

The distinction between bactericidal and bacteriostatic action is relative, in that a bacteriostatic drug may become bactericidal for a sensitive organism. In broad terms, a bactericidal drug makes the growing or replicating cell unstable by inhibiting the formation of structural components. Penicillins, for example, do not affect the synthesis of bacterial proteins, but inhibit the cross-linking of the proteins that form the cell wall (figure 7.4). This creates a bacterial cell that continues to increase in size until it ruptures through the weakened wall. A bacteriostatic drug acts by inhibiting further bacterial growth and replication. Erythromycin, for instance, enters the cell and interferes with the enzymatic pathway for the synthesis of bacterial protein, so stopping further growth. It is wrong to assume that a bactericidal agent must be superior to a bacteriostatic agent in all instances. However, in infections in relatively avascular tissues, e.g. the endocardium, where the patient's own bacterial defences may be less effective, bactericidal agents are superior.

Treatment with Drug Combinations

In the ideal situation, the infecting organism should be identified and its

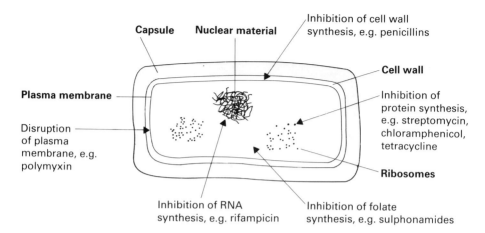

Fig 7.4   Sites of action of antibacterial drugs

antibacterial sensitivity determined in the laboratory before the single optimum therapy is initiated. In practice, any patient with a life-threatening illness requires immediate 'blind' treatment. This treatment, usually with more than one antibacterial, will reflect the most likely causes of infection. To avoid the diagnosis being completely obscured, treatment must be preceded by sample-taking for bacteriological testing.

Combination therapy in specific circumstances can prevent or delay the emergence of bacterial resistance. This type of protocol is virtually mandatory in the treatment of tuberculosis. It has also been shown that, in a burns unit where sepsis is common and cross-infection difficult to prevent, staphylococcal resistance to erythromycin and novobiocin can be delayed when the two antibacterials are used together (Lowbury, 1957).

The most common justification for combination therapy is to achieve synergism, i.e. an overall effect greater than just the additive effect of the two individual drugs. Care must be taken in creating the correct combinations. For example, two bacteriostatic drugs will be simply additive in effect, two bactericidal drugs may be synergistic, but a bacteriostatic drug combined with a bactericidal drug may be antagonistic. This latter situation may arise because bactericidal drugs only kill multiplying bacteria and, if such growth is prevented by a bacteriostatic agent, no killing of organisms can take place. A clear clinical example of this antagonism was demonstrated by much higher mortality in pneumonococcal meningitis observed by Lepper (1951) when chlortetracycline (bacteriostatic) was given in addition to penicillin (bactericidal).

RESISTANCE TO ANTIBACTERIALS

Bacterial resistance is a significant hindrance to the successful treatment of infectious diseases. It is important, too, to remember the ecological balance of the

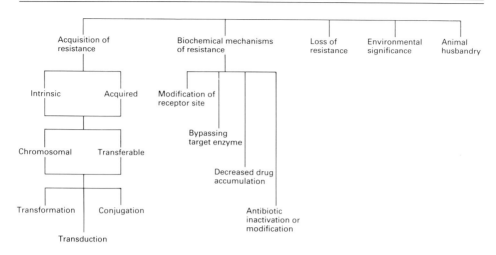

Fig 7.5   Major aspects of bacterial resistance

bacteria with the environment. Figure 7.5 outlines the interlinked aspects of bacterial resistance which will be described in the text.

Acquisition of Resistance

The first scientific paper reporting bacterial adaptation to toxic agents was published by Kassiakoff from the Pasteur Institute in 1887. The significance of resistance for clinical practice was soon appreciated and, indeed, in 1906 Paul Ehrlich attempted to use a single massive dose of arsphenamine in the treatment of syphilis to avoid the resistance that develops with the use of a prolonged course.

Bacterial resistance to antibiotics may be intrinsic or acquired. Intrinsic resistance is associated with a natural property of the organism, while acquired resistance arises either from mutation in sensitive cell populations or by the transfer of resistance from one cell to another.

Intrinsic Resistance

Before an antibiotic can exert its effect it must pass into the cell to reach its target structure. The structure of the bacterial cell envelope is very important in determining penetrability (see figure 2.12).

Gram-negative bacteria are frequently more resistant to antibiotics than are Gram-positive cells. The cell envelopes of the former are structurally and chemically more complex than the latter and demonstrate a sieve effect against large molecules such as vancomycin or rifampicin. The cell wall of a Gram-positive organism, such as *Staphylococcus aureus*, is less bulky and less active as a sieve, but the chemical charge possessed by its component teichoic acid molecules will, literally, repel ionised antibiotic molecules. That the bacterial membrane structure is responsible for the sensitivity or resistance to antibiotics has been further demonstrated by culture experiments. Growing Gram-positive cells in a nutrient-enhanced medium has been shown to increase the lipid content of the bacterial wall so that it becomes more resistant to penicillins (Hugo and Stretton, 1966). Conversely, growth in a nutrient-deficient medium reduces the lipid content and increases the bacterial sensitivity to penicillin and tetracycline (Hugo and Davidson, 1973).

Acquired Resistance

Exposure to antibiotics may select out from the environment a pre-existing resistant mutant. The resistance possessed by this mutant may in turn be transferred to other cells or other bacterial species.

Chromosomal Resistance
The spontaneous appearance of a mutant bacterium resistant to an antibiotic occurs independently of the presence of the drug and at a very low frequency in the range of one in ten million (1 in 10^7) to one in one thousand million (1 in 10^9). However, in the presence of that particular antibiotic, the resistant organism will survive and multiply, so increasing its population of the environment. Clinical problems associated with chromosomal resistance have been encountered with the use of rifampicin, isoniazid and nalidixic acid.

Mutational frequences in bacteria are cumulative. Thus, if the chance of appearance of a mutant resistant to one drug is one in one thousand million (1 in 10^9), the chance of one mutant simultaneously resistant to three drugs is the cube of this, i.e. 1 in 10^{27}. This has practical implications in the treatment of tuberculosis when the administration of three drugs simultaneously diminishes the risk of the emergence of resistant strains of the tubercle bacillus.

Transferable Drug Resistance
Once a drug resistance mutation has arisen, it can be transferred to other bacterial cells by transformation, transduction and conjugation. These mechanisms are discussed in chapter 2.

The discovery of transferable resistance in the 1960s provided the basis for understanding the rapid spread of resistance determinants throughout the bacterial kingdom, and helped to explain why different species seemed to have evolved similar genes coding for resistance.

Biochemical Mechanisms of Bacterial Resistance

Bacteria resist antimicrobial activity by various mechanisms and to varying degrees. Low-level resistance implies that the bacterium may become sensitive to a much increased tissue concentration of a drug, if that can be achieved. High-level resistance implies total resistance, whatever the concentration of the antibiotic.

Modification of the Drug Receptor Site

Many antibacterial drugs act by inhibiting essential enzymes. Resistance may result if an alternative enzyme can be produced which retains affinity for the normal substrate but has relatively little affinity for the inhibiting antibacterial. An example of this type of resistance is provided by the development of sulphonamide resistance by pneumococci. The sulphonamides act by inhibiting an enzyme that converts the substrate para-aminobenzoic acid to essential folic acid. Normally this enzyme has a higher affinity for sulphonamides than for the substrate. Pneumococcal mutants possess a very similar enzyme that has the same affinity for the substrate but with a 100-fold reduction in the affinity for the sulphonamide. Under the environmental pressure of sulphonamide therapy, such mutants will reproduce, resulting in a resistant population.

The protein binding site for an antibiotic is not necessarily an enzyme. For example, streptomycin binds to a segment of the protein-synthesising bacterial ribosome, so the presence of streptomycin causes miscoded proteins to be produced which leads to changes in cellular permeability and respiration and, ultimately, cell death.

An antibiotic can also induce resistance to itself. Erythromycin, which also binds to ribosomal protein, induces a chemical change in the ribosome such that binding is no longer possible.

Bypassing the Target Enzyme

If the primary biosynthetic pathway is inhibited, an increase in the production or activity of enzymes involved in alternative pathways will allow a bypass to be created. Resistance to sulphonamides is effected by the synthesis of a drug-resistant enzyme which substitutes for the normal sulphonamide-sensitive enzyme.

Decreased Drug Accumulation

If insufficient antibiotic reaches its target site within the bacterial cell therapy will not be successful and drug resistance may then be acquired. For instance, tetracycline resistance arises when there is insufficient accumulation inside the cell to maintain the drug's activity.

Antibiotic Inactivation or Modification

Bacterial enzyme systems are capable of inhibiting the activity of antibacterials in a number of ways.

Many similar enzymes have been identified that will destroy the beta-lactam ring structure in antibiotics such as penicillins and cephalosporins. These enzymes are called **beta-lactamases**. A single enzyme can produce resistance to more than one beta-lactam type antibiotic.

Aminoglycoside antibiotics such as gentamicin are not completely inactivated by bacterial enzymes. Modification of the drug's chemical structure is brought about by three bacterial enzymes within the bacterial cell. This structural modification prevents the drug binding to the protein-synthesising ribosome and also interferes with the cellular uptake of unmodified antibiotic.

Chloramphenicol is inactivated by different enzymes in both Gram-positive and Gram-negative bacteria. The enzymes involved are encoded by different genes, and these are usually plasmid transported (see chapter 2).

Loss of Bacterial Resistance

Resistant organisms are at an advantage in the environment containing the drug which they can withstand. On the other side of the coin, some resistant strains are less efficient at survival and replication than non-resistant organisms. In a mixed population of resistant and sensitive organisms in the absence of the drug, the sensitive organisms will, hopefully, outgrow the resistant ones. Resistance may, therefore, be lost when the use of a particular antibacterial is abandoned. This fact has been demonstrated on many occasions in hospitals when withdrawal of a specific antibiotic has eradicated a severe resistance problem.

Environmental Significance of Resistance

Bacterial resistance to antibiotics is a threat to public health throughout the world. Although initially encountered in hospitals, resistant bacteria are now being detected as sources of community acquired infection and as colonisers of human and animal skin, gut and nasal passages. The increased prevalence of resistant bacteria is the direct result of antibiotic overuse and misuse.

Antibiotics in Animal Husbandry

The discussion surrounding the use of antibacterials in animal husbandry is complex as the advantages gained by their use are at least equalled by the disadvantages created. Antibiotics are administered to livestock not only to treat bacterial infections, but also in low concentrations in feed additives as growth-promoting factors. The economic benefits from using less feed per unit of meat produced, and the human benefits from improving the quantity of meat available, have been enormous. An example of the scale of usage of antibiotics in this way is the observation that, in Britain over the five-year period 1963–67, preparations given to animals accounted for 30–40 per cent of the total usage of antibacterials in the country.

There is, however, no doubt that the use of antibacterials in animals leads to the emergence of resistant strains of organisms. The likelihood of transference of these from animals to man depends on the microorganism concerned. If it is incapable of living in man, it is unlikely to transfer resistance to organisms which infect man. For example, drug-resistant *E. coli* transferred from pigs to the bowels of human volunteers was found to be incapable of establishing itself in the human gut, and did not transfer its resistance to native bacteria. However, when the organism is capable of living commensally or pathogenically in man, it may transfer resistance to other organisms or directly cause drug-resistant disease. Such an outbreak has been documented, with drug-resistant *S. typhimurium* being acquired from calves given furazolidone as prophylaxis against infectious diarrhoea (Bowman and Rand, 1985).

The politicoeconomic balance of cheaper, plentiful, but potentially biologically hazardous animal meat when weighed against safer, but more scarce and expensive supplies has led to extensive research into making additive-free farming methods more efficient.

Permanence of Bacterial Resistance

Of great concern is the ability of a bacterial species to become permanently resistant to an antibiotic. This is exemplified by the development of methicillin-resistant *Staphylococcus aureus* (MRSA) (see chapter 10). Methicillin is now little used in humans but is used in laboratories to detect resistance to flucloxacillin. Thus, the term 'methicillin resistance' is used to indicate resistance to flucloxacillin in the clinical situation.

A substantial proportion of *Staph. aureus* organisms possess resistance factors (**R-factors**) on varying sizes of plasmids. Recently isolated, multiply resistant *Staph. aureus* organisms have shown R-determinants to be chromosomally located. Resistance, therefore, does not depend on the transfer of R-factors but is genetically preformed. This situation allows the rapid proliferation of a virulent organism showing, for example, complete resistance to methicillin, streptomycin, gentamicin, amikacin, kanamycin, penicillins (and cephalosporins), erythromycin and fusidic acid.

All MRSA tested so far have been sensitive to vancomycin, and this is the drug of choice in life-threatening infections. Vancomycin is not easy to administer intravenously without inducing serious side-effects such as phlebitis and a shock-like syndrome. It must be infused slowly with care, especially in the presence of renal failure.

ADVERSE REACTIONS TO ANTIBIOTICS

There are no antibiotics in clinical use that are able to damage or destroy the biological dynamics of one living organism, for example bacteria, without exerting some form of adverse effect upon the host. Most adverse effects are understood, so can be avoided or reduced. Ideally, the appropriate antibiotic should be administered at the minimum dose for the minimum length of time.

Direct Chemical Toxicity

Most reported side-effects are due to damage at tissue level. About one third of reactions are allergic in origin, in which the drug molecule or a metabolite binds to a host protein and acts as a **hapten** or trigger molecule for the protein to produce an allergic reaction. The remaining group of reported side-effects appears to include a variety of causes, for example a relative drug overdosage in renal insufficiency or an interaction with another drug.

Prediction of patient susceptibility to side-effects is difficult. It seems that a disposition to atopy, where the patient is over-reactive to environmental or allergenic agents, does not influence either the frequency or severity of adverse drug reactions. On the other hand, it seems that an allergy to drugs acting as haptens is related to a distinct predisposition in the patient. It is manifested by allergic reactions to a number of drugs, or sensitisation after an unusually short time of exposure to a specific agent. In a limited number of these patients, other members of the family show a similar predisposition.

Of the organs and systems involved, the most commonly affected are the gastrointestinal tract (giving rise to nausea, vomiting and diarrhoea) and the skin (causing contact eczema and exanthema). This is probably because of the high cellular turnover of these organs. These reactions are usually of little importance and disappear on withdrawal of the drug concerned. If, however, the drug continues to be administered, severe and even life-threatening reactions may follow. Other systemic reactions, including blood dyscrasias and renal, liver and nervous system damage, occur much less frequently but are potentially much more severe.

Superinfection

Overlong or inappropriate antibacterial use in mild infections may lead to further infective states. Many different organisms live commensally in man, creating harmless microbial flora. Antibacterial treatment of a pathogenic organisms may kill some members of this natural flora. This may free non-susceptible organisms from the competitive balance, and they may multiply to cause a superinfection and secondary disease. It has been estimated that about 2 per cent of patients develop superinfections. Common organisms responsible include staphylococci, proteus, pseudomonas and candida species.

Antibiotic-Associated Colitis

Due to the changes induced in the normal gastrointestinal flora during treatment with broad spectrum oral antibacterials, diarrhoea is found to occur in between 10 and 50 per cent of patients. This adverse effect usually settles following withdrawal of treatment. Occasionally, however, an induced colitis occurs, which may develop during or up to four weeks after treatment. This is a serious complication with copious mucoid and bloody stools, fever, abdominal pain and leucocytosis. The term 'pseudomembraneous colitis' (see chapter 10) describes a condition characterised by plaque-like elevations of the colonic mucosa and, although there have been rare instances of these occurring without an antibiotic association, there is a well-established link between this colitis and excessive antibiotic administration. The cause is an overgrowth of the colonic organism *Clostridium difficile* and the production of its enterotoxin which damages the gut mucosa. Particular association has been made with clindamycin, with estimates of up to 20 per cent of patients developing diarrhoea, and up to 10 per cent of that number proceeding to pseudomembranous colitis. A similar colitis occurs, without the pseudomembranous changes, as a result of enterotoxins produced by a superinfection of *Cl. perfringens*.

Treatment of this severe colitis is to withdraw the causal antibiotic, replace the lost fluids and electrolytes and treat the clostridium infection. Metronidazole, although itself linked with causing pseudomembranous colitis, is used successfully as the preferred first-line therapy. Vancomycin is also very effective but, because of the considerably higher cost per case treated, it should be reserved for any failures of metronidazole therapy.

CONTROL OF ANTIBACTERIAL THERAPY

Antibacterial therapy is controlled by a combination of choosing the appropriate antibiotic for an infection and using the chosen antibiotic correctly.

Control by the Laboratory

There are only a few diseases with a single bacterial cause that is always sensitive to the drug of first choice. The use of antibiotics without bacteriological support or advice must be regarded as guesswork.

The first function of the laboratory is to process the pathological sample supplied, using the appropriate method to encourage growth of microorganisms present and so establish a bacteriological diagnosis (see chapter 6). The assumption that a detected bacterium will be sensitive to a given antibiotic is only true by exception, particularly in the current hospital environment. It is necessary to extend the examination to include determinations of bacterial sensitivity, at least to certain likely antibiotics.

The most useful method that gives a quick and reliable indication of bacterial sensitivity to an antibiotic is based on the diffusion of the antibiotic through a suitable solid medium that supports the growth of the bacterium. A small volume of broth culture or of a resuspended colony from an agar plate is evenly applied to a fresh agar plate and, before its incubation at 37°C, small paper discs onto which a known amount of antibiotic has been dried are firmly applied to the surface. The growth or lack of growth of the culture around the disc, which will gradually release the antibiotic into the agar gel, will give the indication of sensitivity to that

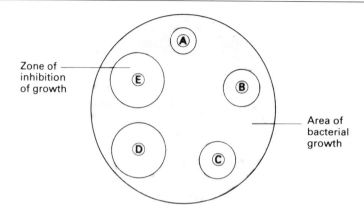

Fig 7.6 Disc sensitivity test. This demonstrates that the organism shows little sensitivity to antibiotic A, moderate sensitivity to drugs B and C, and full sensitivity to antibiotics D and E. Treatment should be with either D or E

antibiotic (figure 7.6). Every laboratory has its own detailed methods of interpreting these **antibiogram tests**. Some laboratories measure the size of the zone of inhibition. A report of 'sensitive' is given when the zone is equal to or larger than that of the control, inferring that the infection should respond to treatment with normal doses. 'Resistant' applies when there is no zone or one of very small radius, implying that clinical response to treatment is unlikely. Other laboratories employ both high and low content discs for each drug and zone sizes are not measured, sensitivity being inferred from observation of presence or absence of growth.

The range of antibiotics used for the disc diffusion test varies according to the source of the sample. For example, after culture of a urine sample from a patient with urinary tract infection, any growth will be tested against a range of antibiotics effective against Gram-negative organisms, which are the likely pathogens.

Factors affecting the results of growth and diffusion tests are many, so great care must be taken to ensure that a standard, reproducible technique is followed. There are many examples of the constituents in the medium affecting certain antibiotics. The addition of blood will reduce the diffusion of antibiotics that are heavily protein bound, such as sodium fusidate. Similarly, the activity of gentamicin varies with the magnesium content of the medium.

Local Antibiotic Policy

To preserve antibiotic effectiveness within a hospital, the local antibiotic policy of use must be adhered to (see chapter 4).

The antibiotic formulary must be educational, highlighting those drugs with which prescribers should be fully familiar. Correct prescribing will ensure effective treatment, avoid unnecessarily induced disease and control costs within this highly expensive field.

The formulary must be local, produced by the hospital or health authority. This will ensure that consideration is given to infections caused by the pathogens found within the actual environment, allowing for local sensitivity patterns and different types of clinical activity. The formulary must remain responsive to changes in bacterial resistance patterns and to the introduction of more effective or appropriate agents.

There are large numbers of antibiotics marketed world-wide, and many have no specific indications. For example, on the UK market there are 14 cephalosporins, all with the same broad indications for clinical use. The problem of which cephalosporin to prescribe may be overcome if the formulary recommends one known to be effective against local pathogens. This information must be represented clearly.

An example of a local antibiotic policy is given in table 7.1 where a representative of the different classes of antibiotics is given, but in such a way that it could be freely available or restricted to specific conditions. As can be seen by looking at the cephalosporin entry, there is one oral formulation and one injectable formulation listed for free prescribing. Any other cephalosporins can only be prescribed on the advice of the bacteriology department. Local policy on surgical prophylaxis and length of treatment is included.

Evaluation of new antibiotics is an integral part of maintaining a formulary that is both useful and credible. Trials of antibiotics tend to be difficult to organise and to

Table 7.1 A suggested antibiotic policy

Group 1 Freely available
Group 2 Available for specific conditions or organisms; held as ward stock on appropriate wards
Group 3 Available only on bacteriological advice and when groups 1 and 2 are unsuitable; not stocked on wards

Limitations on duration of prescriptions – surgical prophylaxis to a maximum of three doses. Prescriptions for treatment are no longer than five days; review and represcription can occur if necessary after that time

Penicillins
Group 1 Oral: Ampicillin   Injectable: Benzylpenicillin
                   Amoxycillin   Ampicillin
                   Flucloxacillin   Flucloxacillin

Group 2 Piperacillin (pseudomonal infections in immunocompromised patients)

Cephalosporins
Group 1 Oral: Cephalexin   Injectable: Cefuroxime

Tetracyclines
Group 1 None

Group 2 Oxytetracycline – dermatology
                   Doxycycline – genitourinary medicine

Aminoglycosides
Group 1 Oral: Neomycin   Injectable: Gentamicin

interpret. For instance, in urinary tract infections relief of symptoms or clinical cure may be obtained without eradicating the bacterial cause. Again, in bacterial endocarditis the blood may become sterile soon after starting antibiotic treatment but prolonged treatment is needed to prevent any relapse. Furthermore, an antibiotic that is very successful in treating a soft tissue infection may show poor effect against the same organism in the urinary tract. Toxic effects of new antibiotics when used in human infections are very difficult to detect in a clinical trial setting, so post-prescribing surveillance must be rigorously carried out.

Establishing an effective antibiotic formulary should be straightforward. It is not difficult to identify the current bacterial population of the particular hospital, the antibiotic sensitivity patterns and the main prescribing areas. A working party or committee should be permanently available to authorise the scope and monitoring of the initial formulary and to evaluate the newer antibiotics. The co-ordination of pharmaceutical, bacteriological, medical and control of infection staff will readily produce a list of antibiotics currently in common use. Frequently, it is seen that 10 or 12 antibiotics will account for 80 to 85 per cent of the prescriptions. Such a common list will become the first approach to the formulary. Additional antibiotics and new products can then be evaluated as above and then allocated either to replace an existing drug or to be held as a reserve preparation to treat bacteria resistant to the recommended antibiotic.

An antibiotic formulary is not restrictive but is rather an educational document promoting the best use of well-understood preparations. Constant sensitivity to changes in clinical practice and flexibility of approach are essential elements in maintaining a well-respected, so well-complied with, formulary.

PRESCRIBING FOR SPECIAL GROUPS

Certain physiological states, e.g. pregnancy, require careful consideration when prescribing medicinal preparations, of which antibiotics are no exception. It is most important to obtain the appropriate information for each specific drug before commencing treatment. Such information can be found in a number of published works (see the further reading list at the end of the chapter), and kept up to date by consulting the local drug information centre.

Prescribing in Pregnancy and Lactation

Pregnant women commonly require antimicrobial therapy, particularly for infections of the upper respiratory and urinary tracts. The pregnant woman, who obviously has a considerable increase in circulating body fluids, will dilute serum concentrations of some antibiotics to as little as half-normal levels. This will not, however, create a clinical problem if the full adult dose is given.

The most serious concern is with placental transfer of the antibacterial to the foetus. On ethical grounds it is impossible to organise a clinical trial intended to assess foetal damage (**teratogenicity**) and, therefore, such evidence is often obtained retrospectively. This has led to a cautious approach to prescribing, with the older, best-known drugs being still the most commonly used, leaving the newer, less well-documented ones for problem situations (table 7.2). The penicillins as a group are described as safe. Sulphonamides, trimethoprim, nitrofurantoin and metronidazole are all probably safe. Although each of these antimicrobials carries a theoretical risk to the foetus based upon the mechanism of action, no evidence of teratogenicity has been found. Antivirals, systemic antifungals, tetracyclines and aminoglycosides have all demonstrated foetal toxicity and should be avoided, although gentamicin can be used if blood levels are monitored.

During lactation, most antibiotics are to be found in the breast milk in low concentrations. In general this is unlikely to affect the baby as only very small quantities will be absorbed, but chloramphenicol and isoniazid are preferably to be avoided. Interestingly, it is reported that metronidazole therapy has an adverse effect on the taste of the milk.

The Neonate

The maturation of tissues and organ function is incomplete until six to 12 months of age. This may result in particular problems for the neonate.

Absorption of an antibiotic depends on both gastric emptying time and gastric acidity. In the infant of under six months of age, gastric emptying time is prolonged and gastric acidity is closer to neutral pH. This combination of immature functions will increase the absorption of, for example, penicillin. Conversely, low skeletal muscle mass and poorly developed blood flow through the tissues will reduce the absorption of intramuscular gentamicin.

Table 7.2   Antimicrobials in pregnancy

Antimicrobial	Safety	Notes
Penicillins	Safe	
Cephalosporins	Safe	
Sulphonamides	Probably safe	Avoid prior to delivery as they increase serum bilirubin
Trimethoprim	Probably safe	Theoretical risk of folate anaemia
Nitrofurantoin	Probably safe	Theoretical risk of haemolysis in rare enzyme condition
Erythromycin stearate	Probably safe	
Metronidazole	Probably safe	Theoretical risk of teratogenicity
Topical antifungals	Probably safe	
Tetracyclines	Avoid	Discolouration and dysplasia of teeth and bones
Aminoglycosides	Avoid, except closely monitored gentamicin	Risk of ototoxicity
Antivirals	Avoid	Teratogenic in animals

Many antibiotics in the blood are bound chemically to plasma protein. In the neonate the level of plasma protein is reduced, so competition with other substances may occur. A drug such as a sulphonamide will displace bilirubin from its carrier protein and may precipitate clinical jaundice.

The immature liver is only able to detoxify and break down drugs at a reduced rate, which will lead to accumulation of the drug and, hence, toxicity. Chloramphenicol is metabolised by the liver and, because of its high toxicity profile, great care must be taken to ensure that only therapeutic serum levels are reached. The kidney does not attain mature function until about six months of age. It is known that aminoglycosides, penicillins and sulphonamides will accumulate, readily reaching toxic levels.

Current awareness of the maturational disadvantages of the neonate has led to conservative prescribing practice. As in the pregnant woman, no clinical trials to estimate toxicity can ethically be carried out. The antibacterials prescribed are usually from a small range of well-documented drugs, and the measurement of actual serum levels attained is carried out wherever possible.

The Child

The older infant and child are said to be 'small-size adults' when considering the body mechanisms by which antibiotics are handled. Antibiotic administration on a dose per unit body weight (mg per kg) basis is generally accepted as safe.

The Elderly

The elderly person undergoes physiological changes that will affect the way in which antibacterials are handled by the body. Blood flow through tissues and organs is diminished, as is the functioning of the kidney and the liver. Resulting from this reduced elimination from the body, the blood concentrations of drugs will be higher, so toxicity reactions may be more common. Antibacterial drugs should be given by mouth as injections may cause sterile abscesses and the resulting tissue break-down may produce pressure sores. As some large tablets or capsules are difficult for the elderly person to swallow, the use of dispersable or liquid formulations of antibiotics will encourage compliance with treatment regimens.

ANTIBIOTICS IN CURRENT USE

Penicillins

The penicillins (table 7.3) show antibacterial activity covering most of the common pathogenic organisms and are probably the least toxic of all antibiotics. Still widely prescribed, their usefulness has diminished because many organisms now produce

Table 7.3 Penicillins

Antibacterial	Indications	Route of administration	Notes
Penicillins			
Benzylpenicillin	Diptheria, tetanus, syphilis, gonorrhoea, meningitis, endocarditis	Parenteral	Bacterial resistance increasing
Phenoxymethylpenicillin (Penicillin V)	Mild, soft tissue infections	Oral, on empty stomach	Bacterial resistance increasing
Broad-spectrum penicillins			
Ampicillin	Pneumonia, bronchitis, urinary tract infections	Parenteral, oral on empty stomach	Resistance increasing, may induce skin rash, diarrhoea
Amoxycillin	As for ampicillin	Parenteral, oral	Well absorbed, good tissue penetration
(Also as augmentin, in combination with the penicillinase inhibitor clavulanic acid)			
Penicillinase-resistant penicillins			
Flucloxacillin	Staphylococcal infections of soft tissue, bone and joint	Parenteral, oral on empty stomach	
Broad-spectrum antipseudomonal penicillins			
Mezocillin	Systemic Gram-negative infections	Parenteral only	
Piperacillin	As mezlocillin, plus anaerobic infections. Superior against pseudomonas	Parenteral only	
Azlocillin	Pseudomonas infections only	Parenteral only	

enzymes (**penicillinases**) which destroy them. For example, in the UK in 1986, 90 per cent of *Staphylococcus aureus* strains were shown to be penicillin-resistant, and 35 per cent of *Escherichia coli* strains were ampicillin-resistant.

The compound clavulanic acid has no significant antibacterial action itself but inhibits the penicillinases produced by a number of bacterial strains. Clavulanic acid has been combined with amoxycillin (as Augmentin) and ticarcillin (as Timentin), which allows antibiotic activity in an otherwise hostile environment.

The most important side-effect of the penicillin group is hypersensitivity, which can cause not only rashes but also fatal anaphylactic reactions. Nausea and diarrhoea during oral treatment are also frequently encountered.

Cephalosporins

This rapidly expanding group of antibiotics (table 7.4) is similar in chemical structure to the penicillins but generally has a wider range of activity and is more

Table 7.4   Cephalosporins

Antibacterial	Indications	Notes
Oral		
Cephalexin, Cephradine	Wide spectrum of moderate infections	First generation; good oral absorption
Cefaclor, Cefadroxil	Second choice in urinary tract infections	First generation; good oral absorption
Parenteral		
Cephazolin, Cephradine, Cefuroxime	Wide spectrum of moderate to severe infections. Surgical prophylaxis	Second generation; more resistant to penicillinases
Cefotaxime, Ceftazidime, Ceftizoxime	Greater anti-Gram-negative activity in severe systemic infections	Third generation; usage may encourage superinfection by resistant organisms

resistant to destruction by bacterial enzymes. The different 'generations' of cephalosporins have been introduced to achieve greater potency and wider-spectrum activity than their predecessors. Unfortunately, their usage can lead to superinfection with resistant bacteria or fungi because of important gaps which exist in the spectrum of each individual cephalosporin. The very high comparative cost of the newer cephalosporins is a further reason for carefully considering their place in routine therapy.

The principal side-effect of the cephalosporins, as with penicillins, is hypersensitivity.

Aminoglycosides

The aminoglycoside group is active against many Gram-negative aerobic organisms and some Gram-positive ones. The spectrum of action can be expanded by combining therapy with other antibiotics, for example a cephalosporin. Aminoglycosides are not normally absorbed from the gut so must be administered selectively for specific sites of infection (see table 7.5).

Table 7.5   Aminoglycosides

Antibacterial	Indications	Notes
Gentamicin	Serious infections caused by Gram-negative bacilli	Parenteral only
Tobramycin, Netilmicin, Amikacin	Reserve for gentamicin-resistant isolates	Lower toxicity; lower resistance rates
Neomycin	Topical use, e.g. otitis externa	Toxicity if absorbed
Streptomycin	Tuberculosis	Resistance develops unless given with other antibiotics

Side-effects are important, particularly oto- and nephrotoxicity. Care must be taken with the dosage, and trough and peak plasma concentrations must be monitored to ensure an effective level of drug without a toxic level being reached. It is also important to avoid the simultaneous administration of drugs which may exhibit similar toxic effects, e.g. ototoxicity may also be caused by diuretics. If an aminoglycoside is used in 'blind' treatment, further antibiotic cover, such as a penicillin or an anti-anaerobic drug, must be given.

Antituberculosis Drugs

The treatment of tuberculosis requires specialised knowledge because of the differing and changing patterns of bacterial resistance to the drugs used, and because of the difficulties in penetrating non-respiratory tissues (see table 7.6). The treatment course is prolonged, comprising an initial phase of eight to 10 weeks using at least three drugs together so that a rapid kill occurs with no drug resistance developing. This is followed by a continuation phase using a pair of effective agents for at least six weeks.

Side-effects are well documented ranging from gastrointestinal to liver function changes, and these may become significant with the prolonged courses of treatment.

Table 7.6 Antituberculosis drugs

Antibacterial	Indications	Notes
Isoniazid	All three drugs are used in initial and continuation phases of treatment	Peripheral neuropathy in high doses
Streptomycin		Parenteral, oto- and renal toxicity
Rifampicin		Gastrointestinal side-effects; liver changes induced. Urine and saliva coloured red
Ethambutol		Visual disturbance
Pyrizinamide	Particularly tuberculous meningitis	Liver damage
Capreomycin Cycloserine	Tuberculosis resistant to the above drugs	Hypersensitivity reactions, neurological effects

Tetracyclines

The widespread use of this broad spectrum group has decreased significantly as a result of increasing bacterial resistance. They still remain effective in certain respiratory, genital tract and dermatological infections. The side-effects are mainly gastrointestinal, but the drugs also deposit in growing bones and teeth and may exacerbate renal failure (see table 7.7).

Table 7.7 Tetracyclines

Antibacterial	Indications	Notes
Tetracycline, Chlortetracycline, Demeclocycline, Oxytetracycline	Respiratory, genital tract (particularly when due to chlamydia) and dermatological infections	Gastrointestinal effects. With care in renal damage, avoid in children
Doxycycline	As above	Safer in poor renal function
Minocycline	Genitourinary tract infections or prophylaxis against meningococci	

Antiparasitic Drugs

Protozoal infections (including malaria) and helminth infections (including intestinal worms) are not infectious diseases commonly seen in the UK. An exception is threadworm, which is successfully treated orally with mebendazole or piperazine, as long as the domestic infective reservoir is sanitised to prevent reinfection and all family members are medicated. Other parasitic infections require specialist advice on prophylaxis and treatment.

Sulphonamides and Trimethoprim

All of the sulphonamide group, and trimethoprim, act by inhibiting closely related stages in bacterial metabolic pathways. This has led to the use of sulphonamides and trimethoprim not only as single agents but also in combination (table 7.8).

Sulphonamides are the oldest systemic antibacterials still in regular use – if only just. Their use is restricted because of the high incidence of resistance and a wide range of minor and major side-effects when compared with other antibiotics. Because of good penetration into the cerebrospinal fluid, parenteral sulphadimidine is occasionally used in prophylaxis in patients with skull fractures to prevent bacterial meningitis.

Trimethoprim has a broad spectrum of activity and distributes very well into the body's tissues and fluids. It causes fewer side-effects than the sulphonamides, and is

Table 7.8 Sulphonamides and trimethoprim

Antibacterial	Indications	Route of administration
Sulphadiazine, Sulphadimidine	Prophylaxis for sensitive meningococcal and urinary tract infections	Oral, parenteral
Trimethoprim	Urinary tract infections, acute and chronic bronchitis	Oral, parenteral
Cotrimoxazole (sulphamethoxazole 5 parts trimethoprim 1 part)	Infections of respiratory, gastrointestinal and urinary tracts	Oral, parenteral

used alone in the treatment of respiratory and urinary tract infections. Unfortunately, resistance appears to be developing, probably by the 'selecting out' of resistant strains.

Combination of a sulphonamide with trimethoprim does seem to improve the effectiveness of both antibacterials, if the organisms are sensitive to both, particularly in some chronic infective conditions. The side-effects of the combinations will be those of the individual components so the combination may have little to offer, on balance, over trimethoprim alone.

Side-effects of the group of drugs range from nausea, vomiting and skin rashes to blood dyscrasias and megaloblastic anaemia. Prolonged treatment courses should be monitored, particularly for haematological toxicity.

Other Antibacterial Agents

(See table 7.9)

Erythromycin has a similar spectrum of activity to penicillin and is used as an alternative in penicillin-allergic patients. In addition, it is active against certain unusual organisms such as mycoplasma, legionella and campylobacter. It is active against many penicillin-resistant staphylococci and genital tract organisms. Side-effects are mainly on the gastrointestinal tract, but the estolate salt of erythromycin may cause cholestatic jaundice after prolonged use.

Clindamycin shows good tissue penetration and activity. It is indicated for staphylococcal bone and joint infections and intra-abdominal sepsis. Its usefulness is, however, restricted by serious side-effects, the most important of which is pseudomembranous colitis. This complication, which may be fatal, is due to a toxin produced by *Clostridium difficile*, an anaerobic organism resistant to many antibiotics (see chapter 10). Although this organism is selected out by many commonly used antibiotics, the condition is more frequently seen with clindamycin treatment.

Chloramphenicol is a potent broad spectrum antibiotic. Because of its potential toxicity, systemic use should be reserved for life-threatening infections, for example, meningitis due to *Haemophilus influenza*, or typhoid fever, although trimethroprim is now used in pregnancy for the latter. Topical application, e.g. for ophthalmic infections, is effective and presents virtually no hazard. Chloramphenicol causes widespread haematological toxicity, prolonged courses or excessive dosages leading to leucopaenia and aplastic anaemia. Irreversible aplastic anaemia, which is not dose-related, occurs very rarely.

Colistin is a non-orally absorbed antibiotic active against Gram-negative organisms, including pseudomonas. Such an activity profile has led to its use in skin infections or for bowel sterilisation in immunocompromised patients. An injectable form is available for intramuscular administration, but is little used because of toxicity. Inhalation administration has been successfully used in treating sensitive bronchitic infections. The side-effects from systemically absorbed colistin are mainly neurological, including vertigo and muscle weakness.

Table 7.9   Other antibacterial agents

Antibacterial	Indications	Route of administration	Notes
Erythromycin	Respiratory and genital tract infections, particularly mycoplasma, legionella and severe campylobacter infections	Oral, intravenous	Alternative to penicillin. Estolate salt toxic to liver if long treatment course
Clindamycin	Staphylococcal bone and tissue infections		Frequently causes pseudomembranous colitis
Chloramphenicol	Systemic use restricted to life-threatening infections. Topical in ophthalmic infections	Oral, parenteral	Severe haematological toxicity. Levels must be monitored
Colistin	Bowel sterilisation; also by inhalation in cystic fibrosis	Not absorbed from oral dose	Neurological toxicity from parenteral administration
Polymixin	Systemic or bladder infections of sensitive Gram-negative organisms	As for colistin	
Sodium fusidate	Penicillin-resistant staphylococci, especially deep tissue and bone	Oral, intravenous, topical	Resistance may develop rapidly
Vancomycin	Systemic: Gram-positive infections resistant to other antibiotics, e.g. MRSA. Oral: Pseudomembranous colitis	Oral and intravenous	Infrequent development of resistance. Nephrotoxic. Sensitivity reaction unless slow infusion
Metronidazole	Surgical and gynaecological anaerobic infections, prophylaxis. Pseudomembranous colitis	Orally and rectally well absorbed; parenteral	
Nitrofurantion	Wide range of urinary tract infections	Oral, requires acidic urine	Gastrointentinal upset can occur
Nalidixic acid	Gram-negative urinary tract infections	Oral	Resistance may develop rapidly Gastrointestinal side-effects
Noxythiolin	Topical bacterial and fungal infections	By instillation to bladder or peritoneum	
Rifampicin	Antituberculosis therapy, also oral prophylaxis against meningococci	Oral, intravenous	

Polymixin has a similar activity and toxicity to colistin. Its use is restricted to intravenous or bladder installation therapy for sensitive infections.

Sodium fusidate (Fucidin) is a highly active, narrow spectrum antibiotic which penetrates well into body tissues, particularly bone. The main indication for use is against penicillin-resistant staphylococci, especially in osteomyelitis. Because resistance may develop during treatment, simultaneous administration of a second anti-staphylococcal antibiotic is essential. Side-effects are mainly gastrointestinal, but reversible changes in liver function may occur.

Vancomycin is effective against most Gram-positive bacteria, including those that are multiply resistant to other antibiotics. Sensitive bacteria do not appear to acquire resistance to vancomycin. This spectrum of activity leads to its main indications for parenteral use, these being the prophylaxis and treatment of endocarditis and central intravenous line and other serious infections caused by multiply resistant staphylococci. It is highly effective by the oral route in the treatment of antibiotic-associated pseudomembranous colitis. As vancomycin is oto- and nephrotoxic and accumulates, it is important to measure plasma concentrations. Slow infusion is essential, as rapid injection may cause a sensitivity reaction of hypotension and a rash over the face and trunk ('red man' syndrome).

Metronidazole was introduced as an antiparasitic drug but is now the drug of choice against anaerobic bacteria. Indications include surgical and gynaecological sepsis in which the activity against the colonic and vaginal anaerobic organisms is very important. Metronidazole is also effective in the treatment of pseudomembranous colitis and, on the grounds of cost and low toxicity alone, should be considered as the first-line drug before vancomycin. It is well absorbed after oral and rectal administration so intravenous infusion should not be unnecessarily used. Side-effects are uncommon but metronidazole is avoided during pregnancy if possible.

Nitrofurantoin is bactericidal to most Gram-positive and Gram-negative urinary tract pathogens, except pseudomonas and proteus species. After administration, therapeutic levels are not reached in the blood, but nitrofurantoin is concentrated in the urine and achieves bactericidal concentrations in acid conditions. Gastrointestinal upset can be avoided by administering larger crystals (macrocrystals) of nitrofurantoin which exhibit a slower gastric solution rate. Resistance to nitrofurantoin develops only rarely.

Nalidixic acid is bactericidal to most Gram-negative urinary tract pathogens except pseudomonas. It is selectively concentrated in the urine, where its activity is not affected by acidity or alkalinity. Resistance may develop rapidly, sometimes within a few days. The most common side-effects are gastrointestinal, but allergic reactions such as urticaria and rashes can occur.

Noxythiolin is a topical antimicrobial and antifungal agent which probably acts by slowly releasing formaldehyde in solution. Indications for its use include treatment of bladder infections by instillation and intraperitoneal use during colonic surgery. Local pain sensation on instillation is relieved by the addition of the local anaesthetic amethocaine.

Antiviral Drugs

Viruses exist within living cells. An antiviral agent therefore has to penetrate the host cell and eradicate the viral material without destroying the host. Until recently such specific therapy was non-existent and treatment was symptomatic, supporting the host while the infection resolved spontaneously. This approach is satisfactory, for example, in viral childhood upper respiratory tract infections. Severe viral infections such as meningitis, or those occurring in an immunocompromised patient, require parenteral treatment where the benefit must be balanced against the toxicity of the drug used (table 7.10). Prophylactic use offers short-term benefit but is not an alternative to immunisation for long-term resistance to infection.

Acyclovir is active against *herpes simplex* and *varicella zoster* viruses. It can be given topically, orally or parenterally. Treatment should be given as early as possible in the illness for the drug to be effective. Renal function must be carefully monitored.

Idoxuridine was, until the recent introduction of acyclovir, the only substance which could administered parenterally to treat systemic herpes infections. Its intravenous use was restricted by severe haematological toxicity, although it is successfully used topically as a cream or a paint formulated to penetrate skin lesions.

Vidarabine has a similar spectrum of activity and toxicity to idoxuridine, although the side-effects are reported to be less intense. It has been used parenterally in the treatment of infection of immunosuppressed patients.

Amantidine is given orally in the prophylaxis of influenza type A infections. It appears to act by inhibiting penetration of the virus into the host cell, and exhibits relatively mild side-effects.

Levamisole and **inosine pranobex** appear to offer some antiviral effect, possibly by stimulating the immunoprotective systems of the host.

Zidovudine (AZT) is used in the treatment of AIDS or ARC (see Chapter 10).

Table 7.10   Antiviral drugs

Antiviral	Indications	Route of administration	Notes
Acyclovir	Systemic and local herpes simplex or varicella zoster viral infections	Oral, topical and slow intravenous infusion	Monitor renal and liver functions
Idoxuridine	Topical herpetic infections	Cream or paint. Highly toxic parenterally	
Vidarabine	Systemic and topical herpetic infections	Cream or slow intra-venous infusion	Monitor renal and liver functions
Amantidine	Prophylaxis of influenza A	Oral	
Levamisole, Inosine pranobex	Systemic and topical herpetic infections	Oral	Monitor renal function
Zidovudine (AZT)	Acquired immune deficiency syndrome (AIDS) or ARC	Oral	Toxic; may cause bone marrow suppression
Alpha interferons	Virus induced tumours, intralesional infections after surgery. Prophylaxis against viral URTI in high-risk patients by short-term intranasal administration	Not absorbed orally, can be given intranasally	Toxicity shown after long-term prophylaxis

Although no evidence on long-term treatment is yet available, it has been shown to suppress the replication of the human immunodeficiency virus (HIV) within the host cell. Unfortunately it is a toxic drug and a number of side-effects are reported, including bone marrow suppression and anaemia.

Alpha interferons are one major group of a complex family of naturally occurring proteins with broad antiviral, cytotoxic and immunomodulating activity. They do not directly destroy virus cells, but stimulate the synthesis of defensive enzyme systems that will damage the virus strand structure or interfere with viral reproduction. Activity has been demonstrated in inhibiting regrowth after surgery of papovavirus-related tumours, and also in reducing the incidence of common viral upper respiratory tract infections following its short-term intranasal prophylactic use. Further research is required to establish the role of alpha interferon in viral infections.

Antifungal Drugs

Fungal infections are frequently associated with a defect in host resistance. This can occur as part of cytotoxic or immunosuppressive therapy, as a 'selecting' effect following antibacterial therapy or as a result of changing a physiological environment, e.g. vaginal hormone balance upset by oral contraceptives. Antifungal treatment (table 7.11) without consideration of potential causative factors will only show a short-term success.

Amphotericin is active against most fungi and yeasts and is probably the most important drug for the treatment of systemic infections. It only penetrates body tissues and fluids to a small degree. Amphotericin exhibits a wide range of frequently occurring toxic effects which restrict its usage.

Table 7.11 Antifungal drugs

Antifungal	Indications	Route of administration	Notes
Amphotericin	Systemic, intestinal and topical fungal infections	Oral, topical, intravenous	High toxicity with i.v. use
Nystatin	Intestinal and topical candidiasis	Oral, topical	
Flucytosine	Systemic yeast infections	Oral, intravenous	Resistance readily develops
Clotrimazole	Topical dermatophyte and yeast infections	Topical, vaginal	
Ketoconazole	Systemic fungal infections. Not as active as amphotericin		Restricted use due to liver toxicity
Miconazole	Systemic and topical fungal infections. Poor results in many systemic infections	Topical, vaginal, intravenous	May be sensitive to i.v. solvent
Griseofulvin	Dermatophyte fungal infections	Oral	Longer term therapy required

Side-effects following intravenous administration include thrombophlebitis at the site of injection, fever, vomiting, hypokalaemia and nephrotoxicity. The dosage must be increased slowly from 250 μg per kg body weight per day up to a maximum of 1.5 mg per kg per day if the patient can tolerate the treatment. Amphotericin is not absorbed orally so is also used to treat or prevent intestinal and topical candidiasis.

Nystatin is not absorbed orally and is too toxic for parenteral use. It is used principally to treat cutaneous and mucocutaneous candidiasis.

Flucytosine is not active against dermatophytes and aspergillus species, but it can be given both orally and parenterally to treat systemic yeast infections. Side-effects are uncommon but, unfortunately, resistance, both primary and secondary, which develops during treatment, is not. This limits the clinical value of flucytosine, at least as a single agent. It is able to penetrate the cerebrospinal fluid and the vitreous humour and, when used in combination with amphotericin, enables the dosage of the latter to be reduced.

Clotrimazole, econazole, ketoconazole and **miconazole** are members of the imidazole group of drugs, which is active against a wide range of fungi and yeasts. The main indication for their use is the treatment of topical infections. They are all absorbed to some degree after oral administration, but only ketoconazole is absorbed to clinical effect. Unfortunately, its use is restricted as fatal liver toxicity has been recorded.

Miconazole can be given by injection, but the solvent required can cause hypersensitivity reactions. Toxic effects from topical application, e.g. to skin or vagina, are minimal.

Griseofulvin is active against the common dermatological fungi. As it is selectively concentrated in keratin, it is the drug of choice for widespread, intractable fungal infections of the skin. To achieve a prolonged effect on newly forming cells, treatment must be continued for several months.

FUTURE DEVELOPMENTS IN ANTIBACTERIAL THERAPY

Current development and research into antibacterial therapy are mainly directed towards overcoming the increasing problems of drug resistance and broadening the spectra of activity. However, development is also taking place into producing narrower spectrum agents with the intention of treating specific pathogens.

Penicillin therapy is vulnerable to the increasing numbers of bacterial strains producing the penicillinase enzymes. Temocillin, currently in trial, shows exceptional stability to penicillinases. It appears to be active against many Gram-negative organisms and to penetrate well into lung, sputum and abdominal tissues.

Enzyme inhibitors similar to clavulanic acid are being developed, so that existing agents may still be used. An example is sulbactam, which is being tested in combination with ampicillin, and has been successfully used in urinary and respiratory tract infections caused by bacteria showing considerable resistance to ampicillin alone.

Cephalosporins are being developed further with the aim of producing relatively low-toxicity, high-potency antibiotics which will show excellent penetration of tissues such as brain and lung and will not induce resistance. The chance of any one antibiotic being 'ideal' is remote, so several new cephalosporins, such as cefathiamidine or cefpimizole, are expected to come into use in the near future.

Two new antibiotics, related to the cephalosporins, are **aztreonam** and **imipenem**. Aztreonam shows specific activity against Gram-negative aerobic bacteria including pseudomonas, does not appear to induce resistance and appears safe for use in patients hypersensitive to beta-lactam antibiotic agents. Imipenem shows an exceptionally broad spectrum of activity, including most anaerobes resistant to other beta-lactam antibiotics. More information about resistance and toxicity will be needed before its place in therapy can be defined.

New **aminoglycosides** are being developed, having a similar activity to gentamicin but with increased potency and greater resistance to destructive bacterial enzymes. Sissomicin is the one most likely to become clinically useful.

Teicoplanin, similar to vancomycin, shows great activity against Gram-positive bacteria including methicillin-resistant *Staphylococcus aureus*. Currently, teicoplanin appears less toxic than vancomycin, which allows it to be given by bolus injection rather than intravenous infusion. It may replace vancomycin eventually, although some strains of staphylococci appear to be resistant to teicoplanin but sensitive to vancomycin.

The **quinolones**, for example ciprofloxacin and norfloxacin, are derivatives of nalidixic acid. They are highly active against a wide range of Gram-negative strains and are also active against chlamydia and legionella. Good penetration of bone and tissue, few side-effects (so far reported), low resistance (to date) and both oral and parenteral presentations are predictors of wide clinical usage in the future.

The life-saving benefits and the not inconsiderable hazards of antimicrobial treatment have been described above. Existing drugs are being used to optimum effect. The retaliatory response of pathogens in the form of resistance, often induced by the use of the antimicrobials themselves, will present a never-ending need for further research and development. Meanwhile, excessive and unnecessary prescribing of antibacterials in both community and hospital must be controlled. Prescribing patterns need to reflect this control and the public needs to be informed why it should not expect unwarranted medication.

If treated with respect, there will be no shortage of effective and safe antimicrobial therapy with which to combat pathogenic diseases, both now and in the future.

References

Bowman W C and Rand M J (1985) *Textbook of Pharmacology*. Oxford: Blackwell.

Hale White W (1892) *Materia Medica*. London: J A Churchill.

Hugo W B and Davidson J R (1973) Effect of cell lipid depletion on *Staphylococcus aureus* and upon its resistance to antimicrobial agents. *Microbios*, **8**: 63–72.

Hugo W B and Stretton R J (1966) The role of cellular lipid in the resistance of Gram-positive bacteria to penicillins. *Journal of General Microbiology*, **42**: 133–138.

Lepper M H and Dowling H F (1951) Treatment of pneumococcic meningitis with penicillin compared with penicillin plus aureomycin. *Archives of Internal Medicine*, **88**: 489.

Lowbury E J L (1957) Chemotherapy for Staphylococcus aureus. Combined use of novobiocin and erythromycin and other methods in the treatment of burns. *Lancet*, **ii**: 305.

Selwyn S (1980) *The Beta-Lactam Antibiotics*. Sevenoaks: Hodder and Stoughton.

Further Reading

Briggs G G, Freeman R K and Yaffe S J (1986) *Drugs in Pregnancy and Lactation*. Baltimore: Williams and Wilkins.

Conrad K A and Bressler R (1982) *Drug Therapy for the Elderly*. St Louis: C V Mosby.

Garrod L P and O'Grady F (1980) *Antibiotic and Chemotherapy*. Edinburgh: Churchill Livingstone.

Hugo W B and Russell A D (1988) *Pharmaceutical Microbiology*. Oxford: Blackwell.

Insley J (ed.) (1986) *A Paediatric Vade-Mecum*. London: Lloyd-Luke.

Kucers A and Bennett N Mck (1987) *The Use of Antibiotics*. London: Heinemann.

Lancet review article compilation (1982) *Good Antimicrobial Prescribing*. London: *The Lancet*.

Wise R (1987) In: *Prescribing in Pregnancy*, ed. Rubin P C. London: British Medical Journal.

Wilson J T (1981) *Drugs in Breast Milk*. Lancaster: MTP Press.

Journal of Antimicrobial Chemotherapy.

Journal of Hospital Infection.

8

Nursing Intervention

Infection control has emerged as a speciality within the past 20 years, although containment of infectious diseases has been practised for centuries (Keen, 1976). A modern, research-based approach to the control and prevention of infection is essential, but this is an area still fraught with fears, some of which are logically inferred and others ill-founded. Microorganisms are invisible to the naked eye and people are often ill-informed about their source and means of spread, which can result in excessive or irrelevant practices. Many of these control activities are not only costly token efforts but can also end up being more hazardous than effective. For example, 25 ml of concentrated iodine may be added to bath water as an infection control measure. Iodine is active at dilutions of 1/10 to 1/100 (NAPP Laboratories, 1985). If the 25 ml are diluted to more than 2.5 l, the solution is too dilute to be an antiseptic – a costly and useless effort (figure 8.1). When the addition of iodine to the water is used as an alternative to cleaning the bath between patients, the practice then becomes an infection hazard.

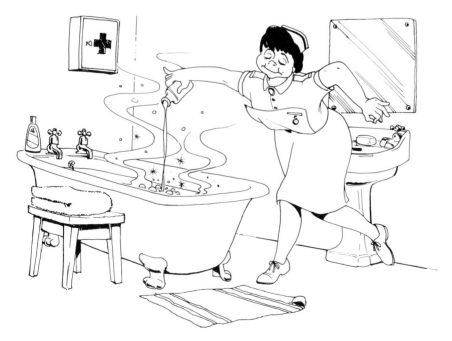

Fig 8.1 Disinfectant in the wrong dilution is not a magic spell

THE CHANGING PICTURE OF INFECTION

Changes that have greatly affected the prevention both of infection and of its spread within the hospital over the last two decades include alterations in:

- The host population
- The problem organism
- The environmental risks

The Host Population

No longer do acute hospital wards house convalescing patients. 'Bed-rest' has been reduced from weeks to days or even hours, and day beds and five-day wards are becoming common (Binnie et al, 1985).

Many previously fatal diseases are now curable or can be controlled. New techniques and treatments allow the patient years or months of good quality life whereas death would have been inevitable only a decade ago. A combination of these factors has resulted in an increased and increasing number of patients whose resistance to infection is considerably reduced by debility, invasive procedures or an immunocompromised state.

The Problem Organism

The change in the host population in hospital has seen the emergence of organisms which were previously considered commensal or non-pathogenic as the problem organisms of the day. They are known collectively as coliforms or Gram-negative rods and include the klebsiella and pseudomonas species and serratia. Referred to as **opportunists** (Swartzberg and Remington, 1979), they appear to have taken advantage of the increased susceptibility of the aforementioned group of patients.

In addition to their emergence as pathogens, many coliforms not only develop resistance to antibiotics but can also pass resistance to each other (see chapter 3). The increased use of antibiotics both for treatment of infection and as a prophylactic measure has enhanced the problem by selecting out resistant strains. During the 1980s, an epidemic strain of *Staphylococcus aureus* has appeared – methicillin-resistant *Staphylococcus aureus* (MRSA) (Ayliffe, 1983) – adding to the current problem organisms and increasing still further the importance of infection control (see chapter 10).

Environmental Risks

The hospital environment would appear to be an ideal situation for the multiplication and spread of microorganisms, with a concentration of susceptible hosts, antibiotic therapy and bacteria. Keeping the microorganisms at a safe level is a constant battle which must be fought conscientiously in order to avoid fatal consequences.

Environmental risk factors include fixtures, fittings and increasingly sophisticated equipment (see chapter 5). The introduction of sheepskins (Jackson, 1983), nebulisers and other items of communal or re-usable equipment, in addition to bedpans, urinals (Hawkins, 1979), wash-bowls (Greaves, 1985) etc., has increased the environmental risks.

The changes mentioned above that have already taken place, as well as the progressive steps in surgery, medicine and nursing, compound infection problems and hazards.

BASIC INFECTION CONTROL NURSING

Infection control is so basic a subject that members of the caring professions may take it for granted. Encouraging members of staff to consider the underlying principles seriously can be challenging and sometimes frustrating. However, this responsibility must be undertaken continuously by those aware of its great importance. Basic infection control measures include:

● The 'Four Cs'
● Hand-washing
● Cleaning
● Drying
● Attention to detail

The 'Four Cs'

Good infection control practice is based on four Cs – care, conscience, common sense and cost-effectiveness.

1. *Care* directed at minimising infection risk should be integral to the patient care delivered by professional carers.

2. A *conscientious* attitude to infection control includes not necessarily omitting all short cuts but ensuring that any short cuts taken do not increase the patient's risk of infection.

3. *Common sense* cannot be assumed. It is, however, the essence of infection control. Practising 'common sense' involves taking a systematic, logical approach to an identified problem. Making time to sit and think is something that members of a physically active profession such as nursing tend to find difficult, and they may even experience guilt when doing so.

4. Successful infection control is also *cost effective*. Not only does it save money, but it also protects the patient from pain, discomfort and worry, and may prevent

extra time being spent in hospital. Planned care will ensure a contribution to the overall cost-effectiveness of the service.

Hand-washing

Hand-washing is the single most important procedure related to infection control and yet the question must be asked, 'Why is such a simple task so arduous?' (Kaplan and McGuckin, 1986). Not only is the frequency of hand-washing important but, more particularly, the thoroughness of hand-washing must also be emphasised.

Informal observations of the general public's hand-washing practices after using public toilets have revealed that, even when hand-washing occurs, few people complete it thoroughly. Despite the fact that some public hand-washing facilities may be far better than those at home or even in some hospitals, the quality of hand-washing leaves much to be desired. Some people only wash their fingertips or one hand. The majority of people perform a palm-rubbing ritual and entirely omit the fingertips, thumbs and the area between the fingers.

Unfortunately, it has been shown that hand-washing in hospitals also leaves much to be desired (Taylor, 1978). Staff must be repeatedly reminded of the importance of good hand-washing techniques (Christensen et al, 1982). The method of washing is of much more importance than the soap or lotion used. Even the most effective or expensive solution will be ineffective if it never gets between fingers or onto the thumbs and fingertips (figure 8.2).

Hands are the most important vehicle of infection. Although this is emphasised in most papers written about infection, we still have to be reminded of it over and over again (Reybrough, 1986). It is also considered to be the key factor in infection control.

Nursing is rapidly becoming research-based, but this research must be applied to nursing practice for its full impact to be felt. Research published by Taylor (1978) highlighted deficiencies in nurses' hand-washing practices which were found to be almost unchanged when the research was repeated six years later by Sedgwick (1984).

Nurses' hands can become very sore after repeated washing, which may account for some measure of reluctance to carry out the procedure dozens of times a day. Careful drying and frequent use of a safely-dispensed hand lotion, supplied in the clinical area, should be encouraged.

Cleaning

Cleanliness in hospital is another major factor in controlling infection. Domestic staff are the key workers, and cleaning the key task.

Environmental cleaning is mainly the responsibility of the domestic manager and his or her staff, although the ward-based domestic worker is, of course, an important member of the ward team. The nurse in charge of the ward must expect and demand ward cleanliness of a high standard. A schedule of activity, acceptable to both nursing and domestic staff, should be drawn up for each ward and department, and a monitoring system should be implemented to ensure that clearly defined standards are maintained.

The domestic department is also responsible for keeping cleaning equipment and machinery free from dirt. Mop heads should be laundered daily and stored dry, and all cleaning cloths and dry mops should be disposable.

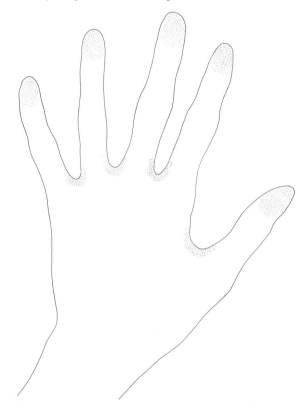

Fig 8.2   Areas commonly overlooked during hand-washing

Any person using equipment should accept responsibility for ensuring that it is cleaned, appropriately disinfected or sterilised and ready for use when next required. The accountable person may enlist the help of others to assist or carry out the procedure itself. Thus, the user's responsibility may end when the item is placed in a central sterile supply department (CSSD) returns container. The need to clean or re-clean dirty, neglected items of equipment in an emergency can be both annoying and dangerous.

The message of the 1960s was 'absence of dust' (Webster and Bowell, 1986), and procedures were adapted to attract rather than disperse dust which was often laden with *Staphlococcus aureus*. This message has been accepted and acted upon to a large extent although, with the emergence of MRSA, its importance must again be addressed.

Drying

In addition to focusing on 'absence of dust', the 1980s have highlighted the importance of 'absence of dregs' (Webster and Bowell, 1986). The major, current problem organisms – the coliforms – thrive in wet places but die rapidly when dried. Containers such as jugs, wash-bowls and mop buckets must be not only thoroughly cleaned and rinsed but also dried. Whether this is physical, using disposable paper towels provided for the purpose, or natural, by placing the equipment in an appropriate position, is unimportant.

An unpublished example which emphasises this occurred during an outbreak of urinary tract infection (caused by a gentamicin-resistant klebsiella species). Environmental screening identified the same causative organisms in the jugs used for emptying closed bladder drainage systems and bed-bath jugs. Cleaning of these had taken place but, after rinsing and emptying, the jugs were stored upright and the dregs which were left in them became an ideal breeding ground for the klebsiella. Urinals and bed-pans were, however, stored vertically in racks and dried naturally; they were found to contain some environmental organisms such as species of bacillus, but no coliform organisms were isolated.

The importance of drying is also relevant to other areas. Bar soap used for hand-washing should be stored on a magnetic holder, not on the side of the basin. Patients' soap should never be wrapped in a face-cloth for storage. Soap dishes should be discouraged, and baths, showers, bidets, etc. should be allowed to dry between users. The isolation room, thoroughly cleaned after discharge of an infected patient, is ready for use again only when it is no longer wet.

Attention to Detail

Attention to detail assumes great importance in the field of infection control. Many factors, however, can contribute considerably to infection; unwashed fingertips, wet face-cloths, dregs in containers, the liquid soap dispenser used continuously without being cleaned and the wet nail brush or wet soap dish, etc. can all create risk of infection.

SPECIFIC INFECTION CONTROL MEASURES

In addition to the basic principles which should always be followed, more formal practices exist to control infection.

Protective Clothing

Special items of clothing can help to protect both the patient and the carer from infection, but their incorrect use results in an additional risk and is also a waste of money (Ayton et al, 1984).

Masks

The hazards related to the use of masks have long been recognised. In most instances, the disadvantages outweigh the advantages, reducing the use of masks to a minimum in most hospitals.

Masks concentrate organisms both on the inside, from the user, and on the outside, from the environment. They cease to function as soon as they become wet. The efficiency of masks depends not only on the material from which they are made, but also on the fact that they may enhance the dispersal of organisms, for example while the wearer is talking or sneezing. (See Ransjo, 1986, for a comparison of the filtering efficiency of different masks under varying circumstances.)

Masks are often pulled down over the chin when not required, and the nose and mouth are seldom covered completely. Following their use, masks should be held by their tapes and discarded; they should not be kept for future service. If used incorrectly, they increase the risk of infection, and many people now consider that masks should be used only in theatre. Some research has suggested that mask-wearing is unnecessary even in theatre, at least by staff not directly involved in the operation (Orr, 1981).

Gowns

Cotton gowns have been traditionally used as a barrier to infection (Babb et al, 1983). On consideration, it is obvious that, although microorganisms are invisible to the naked eye, the spaces between the threads of the cotton gown are not. The usefulness of the cotton gown as a barrier to infection, therefore, appears doubtful, and research has confirmed this. It can be shown that when the cotton gown is wet the passage, or 'strike through', of microorganisms, is enhanced in both directions (Bagshawe et al, 1978).

Where gowns are considered necessary to protect the arms, shoulders and back from splashes of blood, they must be disposable and water-repellent. They should also be made with a complicated microstructure which makes the passage of organisms difficult.

The efficiency of a gown can be further reduced if the user does not fully understand or practise the complex procedure for its use, i.e. hand-washing before and after its removal, careful removal of the gown which avoids pulling the sleeves inside out, careful hanging of the gown (inside the isolation room) to prevent contamination of the inner surface from the outer and disposing of the gown when wet.

For all but a few infection risks, e.g. prevention of contamination by blood-splash from the patient who is hepatitis B e antigen (HBeAg) positive, the gown can be replaced by the plastic apron.

Plastic Aprons

The plastic apron is one of the better items of protective clothing. It is impervious to microorganisms and is cheap and disposable. Even when the inside and outside are clearly marked, it is impossible to store a plastic apron to avoid contamination of the inside from the outside. The re-use of an apron is unsafe practice and to prevent this, aprons should be removed by tearing the waist-ties and neck band (figure 8.3).

Re-use of plastic aprons after spraying with alcohol has been suggested (Lowbury et al, 1981). This would only appear to be cost effective when related to the heavy duty apron made of 50 per cent cotton and 50 per cent polyester. The obvious disadvantage is the possibility of human error occurring during the disinfecting process. Knowledge of the process of and reasons for disinfection, the meticulous implementation of that knowledge by the person performing the procedure and the priority given to its importance, are only a few of the factors which can affect the standard achieved.

Plastic aprons have some disadvantages. They are uncomfortably warm around the waist when worn for a long period of time and the neck band of some brands is very long, leaving the neck area and upper chest uncovered. Their once-only use can also increase the problem of disposal of hospital waste.

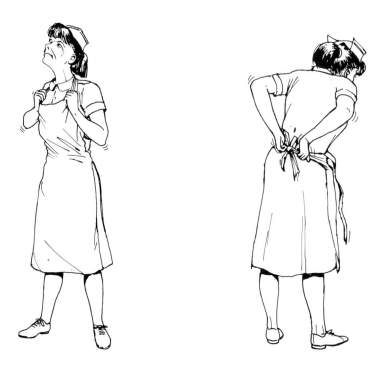

Fig 8.3 Removing a plastic apron by tearing the neck band and waist-tie

Gloves

When used properly, i.e. as a supplement to hand-washing, gloves, both plastic and rubber, are effective items of protective clothing. In the UK, gloves are readily available at a reasonable price and their use for handling excreta and other contaminated material should be encouraged. It must be emphasised that the use of gloves in addition to the process of hand-washing is an added protection, whereas the use of gloves as an alternative to hand-washing may lead to infection (figure 8.4).

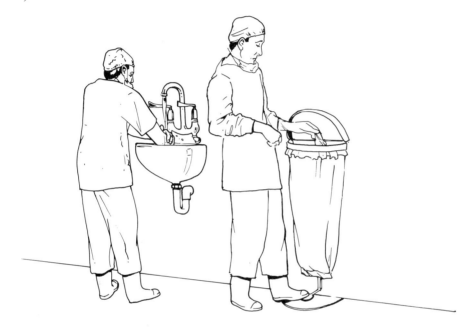

Fig 8.4   Gloves as a protective measure should be used in addition to, not instead of, hand-washing

Overshoes

Microorganisms cannot walk, jump or run; they must 'hitch-hike' from one place to another. When overshoes are worn, microbes can hitch-hike from the floor, where they are relatively harmless, to the outside of the overshoe and, via the user's shoe, to the inside of the overshoe. Removal of the overshoe results in the transfer of microorganisms from the safety of the floor to the potential danger zone of fingers. This situation can easily be overcome by hand-washing, but there may not be hand-washing facilities in the de-gowning area and the wide range of staff and others visiting the area may be unaware of the risks.

Caps

Skin scales can often be seen by the naked eye falling from the scalp and they are consistently colonised by microorganisms (Lennette et al, 1980). Hair covering would, therefore, appear to be appropriate, not only in the operating theatre and food preparation areas where head cover is traditionally worn, but also in clinical areas where invasive procedures involving immunocompromised patients are performed.

Visors and Goggles

The emergence of hepatitis B as a possible infection risk to health-care workers has highlighted the importance of protecting the mucous membranes of the eyes and mouth from blood-splash. Although research to date has shown human immunodeficiency virus (HIV) to be much less infectious than hepatitis B, it is sound practice to extend the procedure for mucous membrane protection to caring for this group of patients. Owing to the difficulty of identifying all HIV positive patients, staff such as dentists, ENT department staff, surgeons and their assistants working in high risk areas should seriously consider their standard policy in relation to protection of the eyes and mouth during high-risk procedures.

There is no point in recommending the use of any item of protective clothing if instructions for its use are not given and understood, and its use supervised. If incorrectly used, even the best protective items can become hazardous.

Disposable Crockery and Cutlery

The use of disposable crockery and cutlery as an aid to infection control is a well-known ritual. This is an expensive exercise which could be considered to be of doubtful cost-effectiveness. For example, the chance of a salmonella infection being conveyed to the kitchen on crockery and cutlery is estimated to be 1 in 5000 (Jackson, 1984). This is reduced to zero when a patient is provided with facilities for hand-washing prior to eating.

One of the few instances in which disposable crockery and cutlery are advisable is when dealing with the patient who is hepatitis B e antigen (HBeAg) positive and bleeding from the mouth following, for example, dental treatment.

Other Specific Measures

Infection control measures also include policies for the disposal of laundry and refuse, sterilisation and disinfection and the use of chemical disinfectants; these topics are all covered in chapter 5.

The success of any infection control measure is dependent on its standard of implementation. Hospital-acquired infection (HAI) resulting from poor infection control practices causes physical and psychological distress for the patient. It is also expensive, estimated to cost the NHS at least £76 million per year (Taylor, 1986), an amount which could be considerably lessened by reducing the incidence of HAI.

The prevention of infection, especially HAI, is one of the foundations of health care and an important indicator of quality of the provision of service (Caddow, 1986).

INDIVIDUALISED PLANNED PATIENT CARE

Prevention of new infection and containment of existing infection is part of total patient care. Infection control measures should not only be prescribed when an obvious problem arises, but also be routinely identified when the patient is assessed. Care, including infection control principles, should be planned and based on an informed application of known facts. This planned care should then be implemented systematically. The success of the care strategy will be evaluated by comparing the actual outcome with preset goals or expected outcomes.

The Problem-Solving Approach

Such an approach is a common, sometimes instinctive reaction to every-day problems. The well-known steps are:

- *Assessing* and identifying the problem
- *Deciding* the best plan of action from alternative options
- *Implementing* the plan of action
- *Evaluating* the outcome

This approach to nursing encompasses not only 'problems' but also 'needs' or 'potential problems'. These 'needs' are related to activities which, due to illness or disability, the patient cannot meet himself. If a need is not met today, it can become a problem tomorrow, so can be seen as a 'potential problem'. For example, the depressed patient who neglects his oral hygiene can quickly develop mouth ulcers or other infectious conditions of the mouth, tongue or gums. Alternatively, needs can be related to existing problems, e.g. the problem of diarrhoea in a patient with salmonellosis is directly related to his need for hygiene, adequate fluid intake and sleep.

Thus, the four main stages of the problem-solving cycle – assessment, planning, implementation and evaluation – can be addressed to both patients' needs and problems.

Assessment

Approximately one in five patients in hospitals in England and Wales has an infection, and nearly half of these infections have been acquired in hospital (Meers et al, 1981). It is, therefore, essential to assess every patient for his 'infection status'.

Two basic patient categories with respect to infection risk are recognised. First is the patient who already has an infection which could in turn spread to others. This patient is a source of infection and is, therefore, a possible 'risk to others'. Second is the patient who, due to some pre-existing condition or aspect of treatment, has acquired a reduced resistance to infection; he is, therefore, 'at risk'. Infection control measures related to these two groups will be discussed below.

Planning

The purpose of the planning stage is to protect the patient from infection. In a 'risk to others' situation, protection must be provided for staff and other patients, while in the 'at risk' situation, protection must be directed towards the 'at risk' patient.

In planning to protect others, the properties of microorganisms (see chapter 2) and the methods and routes of their transmission (see chapter 3) must be understood and applied to the individual situation. Research findings demonstrating the importance of the protective measures, such as the varying aspects of catheter care, can also be considered at this stage (Roe, 1985).

The care plan should be written clearly and succinctly so that it may be easily understood by the patient and all members of the caring team. Care is planned to achieve a specific goal. It is necessary, therefore, to state the goal or expected outcome on the care plan.

Goals can be long term or short term. A long-term goal is, for example, 'John will be able to care for his closed bladder drainage system prior to his discharge'. This may take time to achieve and can be an overwhelming challenge to both staff and patient, leaving all parties frustrated and demoralised. A more acceptable short-term goal may be, 'John will be able to empty his urine bag with minimal assistance within two days', and such a goal is often easier to achieve. Both patient and staff will be encouraged by progress, however small.

At times, even very simple targets can take a long time to reach, suggesting that the goal should be further divided into even shorter 'goal steps' (Binnie, 1985), such as, 'John will be able to drain his urinary drainage bag without contaminating his fingers with urine'. Goals should be patient-centred and must, therefore, reflect the patient's abilities and priorities and be understandable and acceptable to him.

Implementation

Implementation of care is, of necessity, the most important stage of the problem-solving cycle. As far as infection control is concerned, implementation of the plan must incorporate the four Cs described above: care, conscience, common sense and cost-effectiveness. **Careful** thought must be given to priorities related to nursing activities, the methods chosen to administer the care and the time allowed to apply basic infection control measures **conscientiously**. The application of informed **common sense** to this stage of the cycle takes a few minutes' thought, but can assist co-ordination, save unnecessary trips for forgotten items of equipment and result in an overall saving of time. These steps all contribute to **cost-effectiveness**.

A patient with an infection needs to be treated with sensitivity, as he may feel ostracised and stigmatised by his isolation. He may be embarrassed by an offensive discharge or terrified of the implications of an illness such as tuberculosis or HIV infection. Spending time with the patient, especially when isolation is necessary, listening to his problems sympathetically and teaching him about his own safety and that of his family and friends, is all part of the total care given by the nurse. For both the 'risk to others' and the 'at risk' patient in isolation, the nurse who sits with him, holds his hand or touches him may bring the most effective comfort and reassurance (figure 8.5). The route of transmission of the infection and the measures to limit it must, nevertheless, be borne in mind.

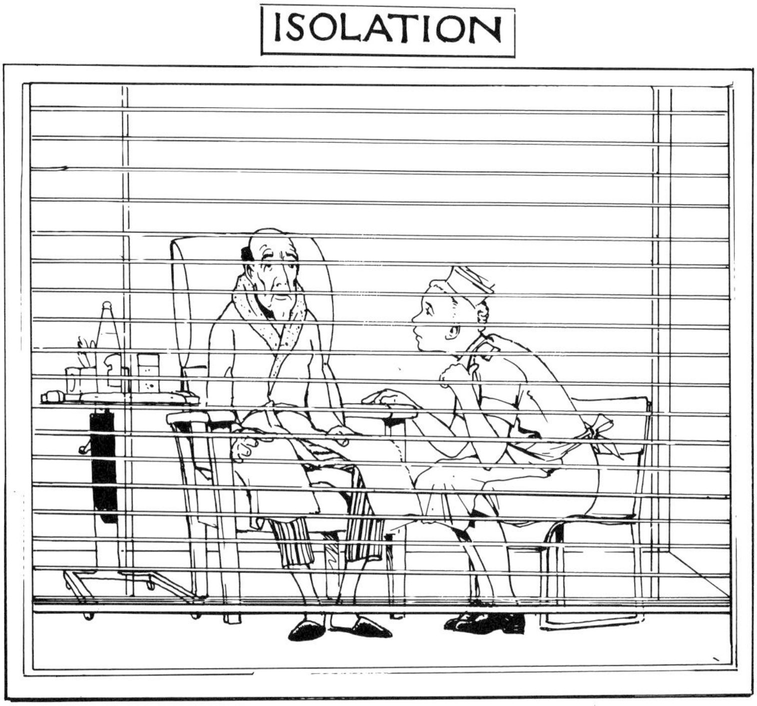

ISOLATION

Fig 8.5   'Isolation' is lonely

Evaluation

The effectiveness of infection control and care can be evaluated by examining the outcome criteria for the situation.

Possibly the best index of success is the lack of microorganisms causing infection and the absence of spread of infection, either within the patient's body or to others.

The number of organisms and their sensitivity to antibiotics can also be a pointer to the patient's condition; for example, the number of organisms in a urine sample can give an indication of whether there is true infection, colonisation or simply contamination of the sample. Sensitivity to antibiotics can assist as a first-line measure in deciding the similarity or otherwise of organisms such as *Staph. aureus*, from two sites or patients. This in turn may suggest cross-infection.

Progress or regress of the patient's symptoms is another useful aspect of evaluation. The patient with a urinary tract infection suffering localised pain when passing urine may progress to being asymptomatic after his fluid intake is increased. Alternatively, he may regress to having generalised symptoms such as pyrexia and malaise, or may even develop bacteraemia (Northwick Park Research Department, 1982).

Progress of healing of a wound is a valuable evaluation measure. Healing may occur by first intention, or evidence of excess inflammation or suppuration may arise.

The Problem-Solving Approach and the Environment

The problem-solving approach can also be used in relation to the environment. Potential risks of infection can be identified, and long- or short-term plans can be prepared with the goal of reducing these risks. Evaluation might include not only routine observation to determine whether or not the plan is being implemented, but also, when appropriate, routine or random environmental sampling to evaluate the success of the plan.

An example of this might be ensuring the cleanliness of wash-bowls. Research has shown that the method of cleaning and storing wash-bowls in a hospital ward can result in their becoming reservoirs for many pathogens (Greaves, 1985). A procedure for care of these items is, therefore, required which includes regular monitoring by the sister-in-charge and random checking by the specialist nurse.

Nursing Models

Assessment and planning in the problem-solving approach are based on the framework of a nursing model, e.g. activities of daily living (Roper, 1985), self-care (Orem, 1980) or adaptation (Riehl and Roy, 1980). Infection control can be incorporated into the framework of any model.

Roper's model lends itself to care of the acutely ill patient with bacteraemia who requires conscientious physical nursing.

Orem's model is an ideal framework for care of the patient whose treatment involves an aseptic procedure, either on a permanent or semipermanent basis, which continues after discharge, e.g. continuous ambulatory peritoneal dialysis (CAPD) or haemodialysis. Here the patient has initial self-care deficits including those of knowledge, skill and motivation. He requires education, psychological help and counselling to overcome these deficits and return him to a self-caring state in which he is safe within the limitations of the procedure.

Roy's adaptation model has many infection control applications, for example, for the patient who has to adapt to a situation of isolation, be it the grim reality of a Trexler tent (Bowell, 1986) or the simple isolation required for a beta-haemolytic streptococcus group A throat infection.

On the other hand, the patient who discovers that he is a carrier of the human immunodeficiency virus (HIV) must adapt not only to the fact that he is a risk to others but also to a new way of life and a future filled with uncertainty and fear. This last example highlights the ripple effects described by Roy in terms of contextual and residual stimuli emanating from an original focus (see Riehl and Roy, 1980).

Each model for nursing views total patient care, patient needs and outcomes from a slightly different angle. The approach of various nursing models can be compared to the experience of people watching a play. Each member of the audience may describe the same drama, but each has a slightly different view depending on his distance, his position in relation to the performance and his own ability to concentrate on and memorise the events. Similarly, an identical script may be differently emphasised by different producers.

Nursing models do, however, go further than this simple analogy as they reflect the model maker's view of man, which is then applied to the patient's illness and his social context. For instance, a self-care model would be inappropriate for an unconscious patient but may be acceptable for someone recovering from an appendicectomy. A common feature of all models is the emphasis on the interplay between the patient's ability to help himself, with guidance, and the therapeutic interventions of the health-care team.

In summary, a model of nursing is an approach or a set of attitudes designed to enable the patient to adapt to his illness and to maximise nursing effectiveness.

CARE FOR THE 'RISK TO OTHERS' PATIENT

For those at high risk of conveying a moderate or severe infection to others, isolation forms a large part of their care. For many years, physical isolation of an infectious patient has been referred to as 'barrier nursing'. This vague term, which means 'nursed within a barrier', implies something different for every health-care worker. The isolation procedure involves far more than providing single patient accommodation within a barrier, so the term 'barrier nursing' should be replaced by **source isolation precautions**.

Some type of barrier is necessary for isolation, but this need not always be a solid partition; indeed, it may be a wall, a curtain or even a chalk line on the floor. Where the infection is contact-spread, i.e. spread by contamination of anything that touches infected material (most frequently the fingers), the best example of which is salmonellosis, the barrier is simply a means of reminding carers, patients and visitors that the infection is present.

Where the infection is airborne, a solid barrier is necessary. Ideally, for source isolation of a patient with an airborne infection to be efficient, an elaborate ventilation system is required (see chapter 5). Without such a system, movement of personnel in and out of the room creates air currents which allow air from the room to escape and disperse microorganisms into other patient-care areas.

Few hospitals can boast sophisticated air extract facilities, so have to adapt their practice to a single room without such equipment. A single room keeps the infected patient at a greater distance from other patients and encourages the dilution of organisms prior to their dispersal. An extractor fan fitted to an outside wall directs expired air away from open wards.

As far as possible, carers should avoid really close contact but, when this would be to the detriment of the patient, such contact should occur but be as transient as possible. As there is no evidence to show that protective clothing reduces the incidence of spread of airborne infection, its use is being progressively abandoned.

The only item which can reasonably be considered is a mask; however, as discussed above, the disadvantages associated with its use usually far outweigh any advantages. One situation where its use can be recommended is when nursing the patient with open pulmonary tuberculosis who requires endobronchial intubation, repeated endobronchial suction, oral hygiene measures or any procedure where frequent close contact is unavoidable. In caring for the patient with open pulmonary TB, the immune status of the carer is, however, the most important consideration. If a mask is worn, the carer must be aware of the 'rules' related to the use and disposal of masks.

It is difficult to isolate effectively patients with childhood diseases and other viral diseases, such as influenza or coryza, as the infectious stage and dissemination of the infection often begin prior to a diagnosis being made. In this situation it is advisable, if possible, to admit to the ward only those who are already immune. The administration of passive immunity to non-immune, high-risk patients may be considered for some viral diseases, for example chickenpox.

Standardisation and Individualisation

Many hospitals in the UK now use a Northwick Park Hospital-style isolation procedure. This system consists of a series of colour-coded cards giving guidelines for specific source isolation precautions (figure 8.6).

When this system was initiated, the instructions on the card were standardised and based on the medical model, isolating the disease rather than the individual (Control of Infection Group, Northwick Park Hospital, 1974). This resulted in a full range of precautions being prescribed for each patient. This approach was

---

Stool-urine-needle isolation

Visitors must report to the nurses' station before entering the room

---

Single room – Necessary: the patient is not to leave the room without medical permission

Aprons or Gowns – Must be worn by all people having contact with the patient or dealing with excreta

Masks – Not necessary

Hands – Must be washed on leaving the room

Gloves – Must be worn by all people likely to become contaminated with excreta

Articles – Must be discarded or disinfected

Collection of blood and other procedures on patients with hepatitis require special measures

---

Fig 8.6   A 'stool–urine–needle' isolation card

acceptable during the 1960s and 1970s when care was task-orientated, but since the introduction of the problem-solving approach to nursing, the system has become outdated. Individualised care is now practised, and in no area of nursing should it be welcomed more than in infection control, particularly with respect to isolation procedures.

The need to individualise infection control recommendations can be illustrated in the following example.

● During one seven-day period, four patients were identified as having an antibiotic-resistant klebsiella species in their urine.

The first patient was an 80-year-old lady, terminally ill following a stroke and with a closed bladder drainage system linked to a urethral catheter. She produced only 200 ml of extremely concentrated, foul-smelling urine per day. It was decided to change the bag daily wearing an apron and gloves, carefully disposing of the urine, urine bag, protective clothing and any bed linen contaminated with urine. After thorough hand-washing, the closed system was left intact for the next 24 hours. As the infection was 'enclosed' within the system, special precautions were seen to be unnecessary between bag changes unless an 'accident' occurred which resulted in leakage of urine.

The second patient, who was also an 80-year-old lady, was confined to bed following a total hip replacement and was incontinent of urine. Precautions were, therefore, necessary every time care which involved handling the patient or her bedding was required.

The third patient, a lady in her 70s, was diabetic and was almost self-caring. A lavatory was designated for her sole use and she was advised on hand-washing techniques.

The fourth lady was elderly and mentally infirm. The sister in the care of the elderly unit was overheard saying, 'That's six beds today already'. While one might be forgiven for assuming that the patient had been incontinent in her own bed six times, what soon became apparent was that, after being incontinent, she left the discomfort of that bed for a nice, new, dry one. She had been incontinent in six different beds that day!

Four women, with the same organism infecting the same system; four patients who would, in the past, all have been classed as 'stool, needle, urine isolation', but presenting four very different problems requiring four different solutions.

The Problem-Solving Approach

As described above, this approach comprises the steps of assessment, planning, implementation and evaluation.

Assessment

The patient may be admitted with a known infection about which the nurse may be informed by the patient himself, the admitting doctor or the patient's general practitioner. Additionally, the nurse's questioning skills and observation, in conjunction with her own knowledge of infection, may lead her to suspect the presence of infection even when it is not reported.

When the patient is diagnosed as having an infection or where there is a strong suspicion of this, the assessment must progress to calculating the degree of risk he may pose to others, i.e. is there a communicable or contagious aspect to the infection? The degree of risk must be ascertained in order to plan appropriate action to suit the individual needs of the patient.

In order to calculate the degree of risk of spreading infection with any accuracy, four aspects must be considered:

1. The site of infection
2. The organism involved
3. The additional risk related to symptoms, treatments and the mental ability of the patient
4. The type of unit or clinical area in which the patient is being nursed

Risk is calculated for each factor as high, medium, low or absent (table 8.1). The score attributed to the 'clinical area involved' will depend on the susceptibility of patients nursed there and the type of infection involved; a urology ward would, for example, have a higher score for multi-resistant urinary tract infection than would a medical ward where few patients were catheterised.

For the sake of objectivity, a scoring system similar to the Norton pressure sore risk scale (Goldstone, 1982) will be used. A score of three points is given for high risk, two points for medium and one point for low risk. Using this system, the degree of risk of transmitting infection from two patients with the same causative organism can be assessed.

● Both George and Gertie (the names they like to be called) have *Staphylococcus aureus* respiratory tract infections. George is a middle-aged man who is the 'life and soul' of the surgical ward. Gertie is an elderly lady with limited mobility who is accommodated in the care of the elderly ward.

   Both patients are playing host to a potentially dangerous pathogen. The infection is in a open site and is being propelled to a varying extent from that site by exhalation, coughing and sneezing. Here the similarity between George and Gertie ends.

   George has a persistent productive cough, filling at least two sputum cups daily. Being the life and soul of the ward, it is difficult to restrain him from visiting the other surgical patients, many of whom allow him a 'peek' at their new wounds (figure 8.7).

   Gertie has little in the way of a cough and is expectorating only minimal amounts. Her mobility limits her to a walk around her bed two or three times a day; otherwise she is confined to bed or to an easy chair.

Table 8.1 Risk assessment for 'risk to others' patients

Site of infection	Organism	Additional risks	Clinical area involved
Respiratory tract	Viruses, e.g. influenza *Staph. aureus* Resistant coliforms Tubercle bacilli	Cough Sputum Mobility	HR MR LR
Gastrointestinal tract	Shigella Salmonella Viruses Pathogenic *E. coli* Campylobacter	Diarrhoea Incontinence Mental state	HR MR LR
Urinary tract	Multiresistant Klebsiella spp. Serratia spp. *E. coli* Pseudomonias spp. Providencia	Bladder drainage Other patients with bladder drainage Incontinence	HR MR LR
Wound/skin	Resistant *Staph. aureus* *Staph. aureus* Haemolytic streptococcus (group A) Resistant coliforms Anaerobes	Discharging wound ● Purulent ● Serous ● Open ● Contained Mental state Shedding of skin scales	HR MR LR
Blood	Hepatitis B virus (shown by HBsAg, HbEAg or Anti-e antibody) HIV	Bleeding ● Splash ● Aerosol ● Open ● Contained Needling Biting by patient	HR MR LR

HR = high risk, MR = medium risk, LR = low risk

When the four weighting categories described in table 8.1 are examined, the degree of risk of George and Gertie for conveying infection is seen to be vastly different (table 8.2). The same organism which is infecting the same site is causing two very different problems.

Planning

After coordinating the information gained at assessment and calculating the degree of risk, an appropriate plan of care is formulated. This plan will incorporate specific precautions aimed at preventing the spread of infection to others. The plan must be simple, clearly written and accessible to all members of the caring team. The answers to four specific questions will determine what relevant nursing activity is prescribed:

● What is infected?
● How does it spread?
● What could be contaminated?
● How can we prevent contamination?

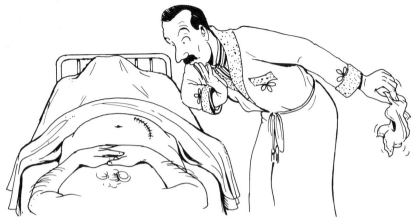

Fig 8.7   George – the life and soul of the ward

The answers to these questions will determine whether or not normal ward practices are adequate, whether specific precautions are necessary and, if they are, what specific precautions are appropriate. Infection control instructions must feature in the care plan as activities prescribed to achieve specific goals related to the infection problem (figure 8.8).

Regrettably, the care plan may not always be conveniently placed for access. Therefore, some sort of identification is necessary to alert staff to the fact that precautions are necessary. Systems range from a coloured sticker informing the reader that advice should be sought from nurse in charge of the ward prior to visiting the patient or a colour-coded standard instruction card to an individualised, printed card with headings that can be completed as appropriate (figure 8.9).

Nursing care plans must be reviewed and evaluated at least daily and infection control precautions need to be amended in accordance with changes in the individual needs of the patient throughout his illness.

Take, for example, the case of Mr Thompson, who was admitted to a medical ward because of 'instability of his diabetes'. He was also known to be a high risk hepatitis B carrier (HBeAg positive). The four key questions were applied to determine the degree of risk of infection to others.

Table 8.2   Risk assessment: George and Gertie

Aspect of infection	George	Gertie
Site	3	3
Organism	3	3
Additional risks		
● Cough	3	1
● Sputum Volume	3	0
● Mobility	3	0
Clinical area involved (see table 8.1)	3	2
Total score	18	9

High risk = 3 points, medium risk = 2 points, low risk = 1 point

Date	Problem	Goal	Activities	Evaluate
1.1.87	Diarrhoea Faeces infected with salmonella	John will understand the need for isolation and the part he can play in preventing the spread of infection. He will not become dehydrated and will maintain morale. His standard of hygiene and comfort will be maintained with minimal embarrassment due to odour	1. Explain the need for isolation and hand-washing. 2. Spend time in John's room when not giving him physical care. 3. Wear a plastic apron when in close contact and gloves when handling excreta. 4. Dispose of excreta carefully. Place refuse in yellow bag and linen in bag in accordance with hospital policy 5. Disinfect bedpan, wash-bowl and Sanichair adequately. 6. Ensure fluid intake of 3–4 L/day. 7. Daily bath or sink wash, hand water after B.O. and when required. 8. Check twice daily for peri-anal excoriation. 9. Discreet use of deodorant.	2.1.87 2.1.87

Fig 8.8   An extract from an individualised care plan

What is infected?

Blood

What could be contaminated?

Needles/syringes
Swabs, disposable drape
Linen
Puncture site
Carer's hands

How does it spread?

Infected blood entering a carer's blood stream via
● a needle prick
● contamination of a break in skin or mucous membrane

How can contamination be prevented?

Safe handling and disposal
Safe disposal as hospital policy
Protect from blood contamination
Apply pressure until bleeding stops
Gloves should be worn during the procedure

Visitors must report to the nurses' station before entering the room	
Complete card in response to questions	What is infected? How does it spread? What could be contaminated? How will we stop it?

Hand-washing

Accommodation

Protective clothing
  Plastic apron
  Gloves
  Other

Disposal of
  Excreta
  Secretions
  Exudate
  Linen
  Refuse
  Other

Fig 8.9   An individualised care card for a person in isolation

As there was no other bleeding problem, the identified risk was related to 'needling'. Precautions were, therefore, limited to times when Mr Thompson was receiving insulin or having a blood sample collected. Between 'needling procedures' no precautions were necessary.

After numerous tests and procedures a diagnosis of laryngeal carcinoma was made and a tracheostomy was performed. Infection control precautions had to be substantially increased. Again, the four questions were applied and additional recommendations were made.

What is infected?
Blood
Blood stained respiratory secretions

How does it spread?
As before

What could be contaminated?
As before
The carer's mucous membranes from blood splash
Theatre instruments

Theatre clothing and linen
Suction apparatus

How can contamination be prevented?
As before
Visor and mask to protect carer's eyes and mouth
Soak open in gluteraldehyde prior to cleaning
Use disposables
Use disposable tubing ⅓; fill suction with 10 per cent hypochlorite (or use a disposable liner)

Implementation

Implementation of the care plan must be careful, conscientious and applied with informed common sense. Any protective clothing that is prescribed must be worn in accordance with the procedure for its use. Staff need to be constantly reminded about hand-washing, and understand when and where this procedure should be carried out. Where applicable, disposable items should be used and, when this is not possible, precise instructions should be given about disinfecting procedures. It is most important to remember that the team involved in the isolation procedure extends beyond nurses and doctors, to medical students, domestic staff, porters, drivers, incinerator operators, staff from the works department, etc. Care must be taken to protect them by ensuring that refuse and laundry are processed safely (Woodcock, 1982; DHSS, 1987), that necessary equipment is available, and that staff are informed and reassured about risks and precautions (see chapter 5).

Evaluation

Evaluation of care given to the patient requiring source isolation may be objective; for example, is the organism still there, have the symptoms improved or worsened, are symptoms confined to the area initially infected or are they generalised, and, most importantly, has infection spread to others? Objectivity of evaluation depends on the way in which the goal is documented. For instance, a patient with hyperpyrexia may have a goal related to the nursing activity prescribed to reduce her temperature, which may be stated subjectively ('Jean will sustain a reduction in temperature') or objectively ('Jean's temperature will be reduced to under x°C in four hours'.)

Frequency of evaluation depends on the aspect of care being considered. Evaluation related to a symptom such as pain and its relief may be carried out half an hour after the problem has been assessed and analgesia given, whereas the evaluation of containment of infectious disease is at least as long as the incubation period.

Evaluation related to infection control will lead to a second assessment, resulting in a rationalisation of the precautions to suit the changing needs of the patient. This results in ensuring safety and cost-effectiveness and also assists the patient's understanding and acceptance of his care.

CARE OF THE 'AT RISK' PATIENT

The term 'reverse barrier nursing', used to describe the precautions taken to protect 'at risk' patients, is even more confusing than the term 'barrier nursing'. The alternative nomenclature, **protective isolation**, is descriptive and now commonly used.

In the past, patients identified as 'at risk' were often those whose maturity, disease or treatment resulted in an immunocompromised state. Although there was a general awareness that other factors contributed to infection risk, these factors were seldom related to the individual patient, nor was their cumulative affect considered.

An appreciation of the mechanism of infection in this group of patients, requires an understanding of:

- The sources and routes of infection (see chapter 3)
- Exogenous and endogenous infection (see chapter 3)
- The immune system (see chapter 3)

Many infections acquired in hospital are exogenous, i.e. contracted from an external source via vehicles such as fingers, equipment, droplets or dust. Endogenous infection, or 'self infection', occurs when organisms spread from one part of the body where they are commensal or beneficial to another where they are pathogenic. Possibly the best example is the infection of the urinary tract by *Escherichia coli*, a commensal of the gastrointestinal tract.

Table 8.3   Risk assessment for identifying 'at risk' patients (The Bowell–Webster risk guide)

General factors	Local factors	Invasive procedures	Drugs	Disease
Age	**Oedema**	**Cannulation**	Cytotoxics	Carcinoma
Very young	Pulmonary	Peripheral		
Very old	Ascites	Central	**Antibiotics**	**Leukaemia**
	Effusion	Parenteral		
Nutrition			**Steroids**	**Aplastic anaemia**
Emaciated	**Ischaemia**	**Catheterisation**		
Thin	Thrombus	Intermittent		**Diabetes mellitus**
Obese	Embolus	Closed drainage		
Dehydrated	Necrosis	Irrigation		**Liver disease**
Mobility	**Skin lesions**	**Surgery**		**Renal disease**
Limited	Trauma	Anaesthesia		
Immobile	Burns	Wound		**AIDS**
Temporary	Ulceration	Wound drainage		
Permanent		Wound/colostomy		
	Foreign body	Implant		
Mental state	Accidental			
Confused	Planned	**Intubation**		
Depressed		Endobronchial suction		
Senile		Humidification		
		Ventilation		
Incontinence				
Urine				
Faeces				
Temporary				
Permanent				
General health				
Weak				
Debilitated				
General hygiene				
Dependence				
Mouth/teeth				
Skin				

The Problem-Solving Approach

Assessment

Individualised assessment will identify 'at risk' patients. A guide to identifying risk factors has been produced to assist nurses in highlighting patients in this category (Webster and Bowell, 1986) and is illustrated in table 8.3. It may be simplified for everyday use by using only the main factors (table 8.4).

The Norton pressure sore risk calculator (Goldstone, 1982), and the scoring system discussed above for the 'risk to others' group of patients, score the degree to which each of a small number of factors contributes to the overall risk. The Bowell–Webster risk assessment is, on the other hand, only a guide. It simply sets out five correlated lists of elements ranging from the major infection hazards to the more minor contributing factors.

Producing an actual figure to denote each factor's relative contribution to the overall risk is difficult as, to produce a comprehensive score, each item in each column requires a separate weighting. Obviously, surgery or a disease such as leukaemia constitutes a risk factor that is far greater than that of age or immobility. However, age, immobility or any other element from the 'general factors' column can considerably increase the patient's risk of infection in the presence of a major factor. Risk factors are easily identified and the size of the problem can be estimated by stating the number of risk factors detected.

For example, Mrs Hornsby, an obese 80-year-old lady, has just undergone surgery following a fractured femur. Retention of urine has necessitated closed bladder drainage, and Mrs Hornsby also has an intravenous infusion in progress. Her 'at risk' assessment identifies these predisposing factors:

- Age
- Obesity
- Surgery
- Intubation
- Foreign body
- Reduced mobility
- Urethral catheter
- Intravenous infusion

Table 8.4   Modified Bowell–Webster risk guide

General factors	Local factors	Invasive procedures	Drugs	Disease
Age	Oedema	Cannulation	Cytotoxics	Carcinoma
Nutrition	Ischaemia	Catheterisation	Antibiotics	Leukaemia
Mobility	Skin lesions	Surgery	Steroids	Anaemia
Mental state	Foreign body	Intubation		Diabetes
Incontinence				Liver disease
General health				Renal disease
General hygiene				AIDS

(Tables 8.3 and 8.4 are reproduced by kind permission of *Nursing Times* where they first appeared in the Infection Control Supplement, 4 June 1986.)

Mrs Hornsby's score is 8. This would be further increased by additional postoperative factors such as confusion, oedema and weakness.

In contrast Malcolm, a young executive, has returned from theatre following an appendicectomy. Malcolm's 'at risk' assessment identifies these predisposing factors:

● Surgery
● Intubation

Malcolm's score is 2.

A mathematical model to assist in the accurate calculation of infection risk for each individual has been described by Collins (1986). The computations involved are complex which may limit the model's suitability for everyday use.

Planning

Prevention of exogenous infection begins by identifying vehicles which could be employed by the organisms to 'hitch-hike' to a susceptible site. These vehicles include:

● People
● The environment
● Reusable equipment (linen, crockery, bedpans and urinals)
● Invasive procedures
● Food

Prevention of endogenous infection begins with the awareness of its possibility. The safest place for a person at risk of such an infection to be is in his own home (see chapter 4). Prevention of infection in hospital requires a ward environment free from antibiotic-resistant organisms. Patients quickly become colonised with hospital organisms (Shanson, 1982). Allowing resistant organisms to flourish in the environment may result in their colonising patients, which may be dangerous.

Relevant precautions differ greatly for individual patients, and from hospital to hospital. Patients requiring physical isolation will benefit from filtered air under positive pressure which ensures the flow of air from 'clean' to contaminated areas. An extreme set of precautions for intensive protection may be prescribed in, for example, the patient with neutropaenia who is undergoing bone marrow transplantation. The patient is nursed in a specially constructed room providing a Trexler tent similar to that described for source isolation of exotic diseases (Bowell, 1986), where only the patient is isolated. An alternative environment is a room with laminar flow ventilation and an airlock entrance. The latter system involves both patient and staff in the isolation procedure. The staff are able to give direct care, having showered and dressed completely in protective clothing. Elaborate care will be wasted, however, if the patient still has millions of microorganisms in his gastrointestinal tract which could become a source of endogenous infection. Precautions must therefore include 'gut sterilisation' and the provision of 'ultra-clean food' containing no pathogens. This extreme isolation technique may induce intolerable psychological problems for the patient.

A patient who has undergone an invasive procedure is also 'at risk'. This fact is sometimes not well understood by staff; for example, inadequate aseptic care of the intravenous infusion site and poor aseptic care of a closed bladder drainage system can still occur despite every attempt at education.

Using Roper's model as a framework, problems of infection can be described under 'maintenance of safety'. An example of part of a care plan for an immunosuppressed patient is given in figure 8.10.

Implementation

Implementation of the plan will be based on the principles of informed, conscientious care. Many patients at increased risk of infection may be safely nursed in the open ward without specific isolation precautions. This emphasises the importance of the basic infection control standards described at the beginning of the chapter.

The positioning of the patient in the ward is important for the control of infection. When allocating the bed and bed space, facilities required for nursing the patient and the position of any other patients suffering from infection must be considered. Research has shown, for example, that a catheterised patient is most at risk of infection in the bed directly opposite or next to another catheterised patient (Northwick Park Research Department, 1982).

Staff caring for the patient should be free from infection and, where possible, they should be limited to caring for infection-free patients. Where nurses find they have to care for both 'risk to others' and 'at risk' patients, the highest standard of implementation of infection control measures, especially hand-washing, is paramount.

Date	Problem	Goal	Nursing activity	Evaluation
1.1.87	Maintenance of safety 1. Inability to resist infection due to immuno-compromised state	Jean will suffer no infection episode during her stay in hospital	1. Impeccable hand-washing prior to handling 2. Educate patient about handwashing 3. Nurse in a single room with: a. extractor fan b. door closed 4. Use of disposable equipment Safely disinfect reusable equipment 5. Daily linen change 6. Other, e.g. psychological care	2.1.87

Fig 8.10 Part of a care plan for an immunosuppressed patient

Evaluation

Evaluation of the high-risk patient from an infection point of view is fairly simple. The patient is either free of infection or he is not. The nurse may recognise a change in the patient in terms of his colour, increasing malaise, odour etc., which may signal an imminent episode of infection. An evaluation which includes this type of reassessment, observation and sensitivity will initiate further nursing activity, such as recording the pulse and temperature more frequently, obtaining a specimen for the laboratory or alerting the medical staff.

HOLISTIC CARE

All patients need holistic care, i.e. consideration of the whole person, but this is particularly important for the patient who is physically isolated. Holistic care has physical, psychological and social aspects.

Physical Care

Isolation of patients is rare in most general wards. When the need for it arises, it may be met with fear or lack of confidence by the health-care team. Routinely assessing the infection status of every patient could help to overcome the apprehension associated with the isolation procedure. If infection and its prevention were given the priority they deserve, the necessary isolation procedures could be automatically incorporated into an individualised plan of care.

Physical care includes both the administration of the specific treatment prescribed by the medical staff and the symptomatic treatment which is frequently initiated by nurses. Symptomatic treatment is often required for pain, nausea, hyperpyrexia or headache. Nursing measures such as a cold compress for a headache, turning a hot pillow, providing ice-cold water to drink or changing a patient's position can often be as successful as symptomatic drug therapy.

Psychological and Social Care

Patients in isolation often, for very good reasons, feel lonely and afraid, so psychological and emotional aspects of care are vital. It is essential to spend time with the patient, listening to voiced anxieties, explaining the specific infection problem and giving reasons for the isolation precautions. The patient and his relatives should be involved in all infection control activities (see chapter 5).

Informed discretion must be applied to measures necessary to protect the nurse who is visiting the patient 'for a chat' when no physical care is required. There is often no need to use protective clothing during such a social visit, especially with contact-spread infections such as salmonellosis. In such a case, the nurse would avoid sitting on the bed and must hand-wash when leaving the room but, unless physical care becomes necessary, no special precautions are required.

SUMMARY

Infection control can never be divorced from ward management and patient care. Awareness of actual and potential infection hazards is absolutely essential if a reduction in hospital-acquired infection is to be achieved.

The nurse who, by using a systematic approach, is able to recognise potential problems and proceeds to plan appropriate prevention and control measures is a tremendous asset to both the caring team and the patient. A sensitive and complete individualised patient care plan will reflect an understanding of microbial behaviour and an awareness of current research.

Instructions can be given, knowledge can be disseminated and education offered, but it is the responsibility of each individual member of staff to obey instructions and demonstrate wisdom by assimilating and applying the knowledge received. Practices are as efficient as the practitioner and they are the responsibility of every member of the health-care team.

References

Ayliffe G A J (1983) Methicillin resistant *Staphylococcus aureus. Journal of Hospital Infection*, **4**(4): 372–373.

Ayton M, Babb J, Mackintosh C and Maloney M (1984) *Report of the Infection Control Nurses Association Working Party on Ward Protective Clothing*. London: ICNA.

Babb J R, Davies J G and Ayliffe G A J (1983) Contamination of protective clothing and nurses' uniforms in an isolation ward. *Journal of Hospital Infection*, **4**(2): 149–157.

Bagshawe K D, Blowers R and Lidwell O M (1978) Isolating patients in hospital to control infection, IV: Nursing procedures. *British Medical Journal*, **2**: 808–811.

Binnie A, Bond S, Law G, Lowe K, Pearson A, Roberts R, Tierney A, Vaughan B (1985) *A Systematic Approach to Nursing Care*. Milton Keynes: The Open University Press.

Bowell E (1986) Nursing the isolated patient: Lassa fever. *Nursing Times*, **82**(38), *Journal of Infection Control*, pp. 72–81.

Caddow P (1986) Questions on quality. *Nursing Times*, **81**(28): 42–43.

Christensen G D, Korones S B, Reed L, Bulley R, McLaughlan B and Bisno A L (1982) Epidemic *Serratia marcescens* in a neonatal intensive care unit. *Infection Control*, **3**(2): 127–133.

Collins B (1986) A ward mathematical model. In: *Infection Control Year Book 1987*, pp. 173–176. Cambridge: CMA Medical Data Ltd, for the Infection Control Nurses Association.

Control of Infection Group, Northwick Park Hospital and Clinical Research Centre (1974) Isolation system for general hospitals. *British Medical Journal*, **6**(ii): 41–46.

Department of Health and Social Security (1987) *Hospital Laundry Arrangements for Used and Infected Linen*. London: HMSO.

Goldstone L A (1982) The Norton score: an early warning of pressure sores? *Journal of Advanced Nursing*, **7**: 419–426.

Greaves A (1985) 'We'll just freshen you up dear . . .' *Nursing Times*, **81**(10), *Journal of Infection Control Nursing*, pp. 3–8.

Hawkins C M (1979) A survey of systems in use for disposal/disinfection of bedpans and associated equipment. *Nursing Times*, Contact, **12**: 13–16.

Jackson J (1983) Sheepskins – a potential hazard. *Nursing Times*, **79**(18), *Journal of Infection Control Nursing*, pp. 41–45.

Jackson M M (1984) From ritual to reason. *American Journal of Infection Control*, **12**(4): 213–220.

Kaplan L M and McGuckin M (1986) Increasing handwashing compliance with more accessible sinks. *Infection Control*, **7**(8): 408–410.

Keen H, Jarrett J, Levy A M and Elik P (1976) *Triumphs of Medicine*. London: Paul Elek.

Lennette E H et al (1980) *Manual of Clinical Microbiology*, 3rd edn. Washington DC: American Society of Microbiology.

Lowbury E J L, Ayliffe G A J, Geddes A M and Williams J D (1981) *Control of Hospital Infection*, 2nd edn. London: Chapman and Hall.

Meers P D, Ayliffe G A J, Emmerson A M, Leigh D A, Mayon-White R T, Mackintosh C A and Strong J L (1981) Report on the national survey of infection in hospitals, 1980. *Journal of Hospital Infection*, **2**: supplement.

Napp Laboratories (1985) *The Importance of Production Formulation to the Microbicidal Efficacy of Povidone-Iodine Solutions*. Cambridge: Haff Laboratories.

Northwick Park Hospital Research Department (1982) Proceedings of a Conference held at Northwick Park Hospital, Middlesex.

Orem D E (1980) *Nursing: Concepts of Practice*. New York: McGraw Hill.

Orr N W M (1981) Is a mask necessary in an operating theatre? *Annals of the Royal College of Surgeons of England*, **63**: 930–932.

Ransjo U (1986) Masks: a ward investigation and review of the literature. *Journal of Hospital Infection*, **7**(3): 283–293.

Reybrough G (1986) Handwashing and hand disinfection. *Journal of Hospital Infection*, **8**(1): 5–23.

Riehl J P and Roy C (1980) *Conceptual Models for Nursing Practice*, 2nd edn. New York: Norwalk Appleton Century Crofts.

Roe B (1985) Catheter care, an overall view. *Internal Journal of Nursing Studies*, **22**(1): 45–46.

Roper N, Logan W W and Tierney A J (1985) *The Elements of Nursing*, 2nd edn. Edinburgh: Churchill Livingstone.

Sedgwick J (1984) Handwashing in hospital wards. *Nursing Times*, **80**(20), *Journal of Infection Control Nursing*, pp. 64–67.

Shanson D C (1982) *Microbiology in Clinical Practice*. Bristol: John Wright.

Swartzberg J E and Remington J S (1979) In: *Hospital Infections*, eds Bennett J V and Brachman H. Boston: Little Brown.

Taylor L (1986) Hospital acquired infections. *Self Health*, **11**: 8–9.

Taylor L J (1987) An evaluation of handwashing techniques, 1 and 2. *Nursing Times*, **74**(2): 54, **74**(3): 108–110.

Webster O and Bowell E (1986) Thinking prevention. *Nursing Times*, **82**(23), *Journal of Infection Control Nursing*, pp. 68–74.

Woodcock P (1982) *The Safe Disposal of Clinical Waste*. London: HMSO.

Further Reading

Marks J (1983) Salt in the bathwater. Letter to the Editor. *Nursing Times*, **79**(30): 7.

Watson M (1984) Salt in the bath. *Nursing Times*, Occasional Paper, **80**(19): 57–59.

9

National and International

Epidemiology

The harassed staff on a busy surgical ward might well be sceptical about the workings of grandiose international authorities like the World Health Organisation (WHO). This chapter attempts to give an overview of some of the major health care bodies and to explain their relevance to everyone engaged in promoting health and caring for the ill.

THE WORLD HEALTH ORGANISATION

The WHO administers international health regulations to minimise the spread of disease. Co-operation is needed between the responsible nations for these regulations to be effective. Plague, cholera and yellow fever are all dealt with by these regulations, as are the disinfection of aircraft and the de-ratting of ships. An example of successful international co-operation in combating disease is the eradication of smallpox.

The officers of the WHO are responsible for assisting individual nations to collect information on infectious diseases and to co-ordinate the dissemination of this data. Their aim is to improve health by ensuring that countries co-operate with each other so that the most effective and rational approach is used to prevent and control the spread of infection.

The WHO also acts as a resource for health workers by collecting, consolidating and publishing epidemiological information from different countries. This is obviously no simple task. Even within the same health district variations can be found in the way diseases are notified, investigated, diagnosed and reported. The variations between different countries are even greater, and the WHO attempts to present the information it receives in a coherent and comprehensive way.

The staff of the WHO provide technical advice and training facilities to help countries to standardise their methodology and reporting systems. They offer reference material to inform and update health-care workers, and can help to implement surveillance programmes.

Epidemiological information needs continuous interpretation as disease patterns change and more people travel to new countries. For example, in Europe, there is constant movement between northern (wealthier) residents and those from the poorer south, as the northerners migrate south for holidays in ever increasing numbers, and southerners flock to northern countries in search of work. As a result, groups develop such as the Turkish 'Gastarbeiten' who now form a significant proportion of the population of many cities in West Germany.

Industrialised countries have reduced the numbers of people suffering from some microbial diseases, e.g. tuberculosis, typhoid, measles, malaria and diptheria, by improving socioeconomic conditions and by immunisation programmes and prophylactic schemes. However, the emergence of new diseases bears out the prophetic works of Professor Lucas, published in *Public Health in Europe*, ten years before the Western world heard of acquired immune deficiency syndrome (AIDS):

●   'Because of the great successes which have been achieved, it is perhaps tempting to assume that the problem of communicable diseases is virtually solved and that victory is just around the corner. There is, however, ample evidence that such complacency and a premature relaxation of effort in the attack against communicable diseases could lead to disappointing setbacks or even disastrous consequences.' (Lucas, 1974)

The WHO also offers blueprints for the role of public health laboratories in the surveillance and control of infectious diseases. Although many 'old' diseases appear to be dwindling, ultimate effective control can only be maintained by networks of efficient public health laboratories. Competent clinical management and prevention policies are essential prerequisites for the control of communicable disease. These can support national and international surveillance programmes in order to help national health authorities to make national policy decisions for the promotion of health. The WHO can assist public health activities with relevant research, and advise on standardisation to improve the quality of work. Recent technical achievements and discoveries can be publicised efficiently, and follow-up of the spread of aetiological agents can be co-ordinated so that a coherent and effective response can be made.

One of the best known WHO projects is the campaign to eradicate malaria throughout the world. It has had both spectacular successes and crushing defeats. Area and regional programmes were devised and four phases identified:

●   **Preparatory**, for surveillance and training
●   **Active**, when all habitations were sprayed with insecticide two or three times a year for four years
●   **Consolidation**, with surveillance and blood-sampling of the local population until no new case had appeared for three years
●   **Maintenance**, to guard against the importation of malaria from another part of the world

This campaign has removed malaria from continental Europe, the USA and various other parts of the world. However, in other places, progress has been poor because of resistance to the insecticide or to drugs used to treat the disease, or because of lack of co-operation from local people whose cultural needs have not been understood. For example, in the Phillipines, farmers cleared areas of virgin forest to create more arable land during the control phase of the campaign thus creating new mosquito breeding grounds, even though the Phillipinos' health had benefited from the scheme (Acheson and Spencer, 1984).

NATIONAL PROJECTS

In Britain, responsibility for the prevention, control and treatment of communicable diseases is shared between the Government, the National Health Service (NHS) and local authorities; their mutual co-operation is essential.

The Department of Health has overall responsibility for national policy matters relating to communicable diseases. It ensures that adequate and appropriate hospital services are available and supervises immunisation uptake levels at all times. It is also responsible for maintaining international communication networks (e.g. through the WHO) to deal with infectious disease matters.

LOCAL INITIATIVES

Local government district councils (local authorities) have a legal responsibility to control notifiable disease within their boundaries (table 9.1). They appoint community physicians (medical officers for environmental health, MOEHs) who are employed by health authorities to be responsible for the control of infectious diseases within their boundaries. The health authority itself has a broad duty to prevent disease, including communicable diseases. The MOEH liaises closely with the district council's chief environmental health officer to control outbreaks of notifiable disease.

In Britain, most people suffering from communicable diseases are treated at home by the primary care team. The general practitioner (GP) has key responsibility for care.

Table 9.1 Notifiable diseases in England and Wales 1987

Anthrax	Paratyphoid fever
Cholera	Plague
Diptheria	Poliomyelitis (acute)
Dysentery	Rabies
Encephalitis (acute)	Relapsing fever
Food poisoning	Scarlet fever
Infective jaundice	Smallpox
Lassa fever	Tetanus
Leptospirosis	Tuberculosis
Leprosy	Typhoid fever
Malaria	Typhus fever
Marburg disease	Viral haemorrhagic fever
Measles	Whooping cough
Meningitis (acute)	Yellow fever
Ophthalmia neonatorum	

HOSPITAL SERVICES

People who are seriously ill will, of course, be referred to hospital consultants who are advised by the senior professional staff of the infection control team (see chapter 5). They are responsible for reviewing, reporting and treating outbreaks of infection as well as monitoring standards, for example, by collating statistics on neonatal or postoperative infections. They have a wide remit for educating other staff, ensuring that good practices are followed and that services and equipment are used appropriately and efficiently. A great deal of psychological skill is essential when advising fellow professionals on the quality of their care, in order to retain goodwill and co-operation.

Large isolation hospitals are no longer necessary, but most district hospitals have the facility to care for patients needing isolation. Some special hospitals, such as Coppetts Wood in London, still exist to manage infectious diseases like Lassa fever and Marburg disease. These have highly trained staff and a range of equipment needed for the individual's safe management and care.

THE PUBLIC HEALTH LABORATORY SERVICE

The Public Health Laboratory Service (PHLS) plays a key role in monitoring and controlling communicable disease. Originally set up to cope with emergencies anticipated in the Second World War, it has developed into a permanent and invaluable establishment, under the aegis of the Secretary of State for Health. The headquarters are in Colindale, London, with over 50 local and regional laboratories in other parts of the country.

These laboratories undertake microbiological investigations of suspect matter when an outbreak of infectious disease occurs, and also provide a routine sampling service (Donaldson and Donaldson, 1983). They work closely with NHS microbiological services.

THE COMMUNICABLE DISEASE SURVEILLANCE CENTRE

Attached to the PHLS at Colindale is the Communicable Disease Surveillance Centre (CDSC), an infectious disease monitoring unit and a resource centre for community physicians, environmental health officers, clinicians and others responsible for infection control. It is one of the specialist units of PHLS.

The CDSC was established on 1 January 1977 to provide epidemiological assistance and co-ordination in communicable disease control for public health authorities in England and Wales (Galbraith and Young, 1980). This function was previously supplied by medical officers of the DHSS. The CDSC now acts on behalf of the Chief Medical Officers for England and Wales.

As well as co-ordinating education programmes and maintaining a first-class

Table 9.2 Communicable disease surveillance objectives

● Early detection of changes in disease patterns in the population so that rapid preventive action may be taken

● Monitoring long-term trends in disease and infection to assess the need for intervention

● Evaluation of preventive measures

● Provision of information to clinicians about prevalent infections

● Collation of data on rare diseases

● Early recognition of 'new' diseases

(From Galbraith, 1986. Reproduced by kind permission of
Midwife, Health Visitor and Community Nurse.)

library service, the CDSC produces the weekly 'Communicable Disease Report', which lists and analyses instances of infectious disease in England and Wales. CDSC also offers advice and help with the field investigation and control of communicable disease. The Centre has national responsibilities without any executive powers, just as local authorities have legal jurisdiction over the control of infection. It undertakes national surveillance and can deploy specialist community physicians where they are needed (Galbraith, 1982).

The surveillance function of the CDSC (table 9.2) depends on three factors:

1. The systematic collection of data
2. Consolidation and analysis of the collected data
3. Dissemination of information by epidemiological reports

Local experts interpret the information (Raska, 1969) and decide which course of action is needed. The CDSC can guide them in taking this decision and assist in its implementation. Staff from the CDSC are also involved in evaluating the process and feeding back reports from other centres. Thus the cycle is completed (figure 9.1). The methodology is shown in table 9.3.

The Communicable Disease Surveillance Centre is staffed by specialist community physicians with scientific and administrative back-up staff, including a control of infection nurse. Staff are responsible, via the PHLS board, to the Secretary of State for Health. A 24-hour on-call service is provided by the physicians for emergency cover. Specialist training is offered for doctors, and teaching material is available from the CDSC for any other interested parties.

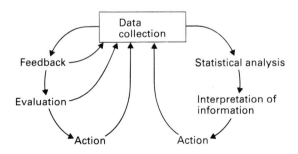

Fig 9.1 The process of surveillance

In addition to the frequency registered by the monitoring service supplied by the CDSC, a record is kept of all notifiable diseases by the Office of Population Censuses and Surveys (OPCS). This is published in the 'Registrar General's Week Return for England and Wales'. The 'Return', which is sent to all district medical officers (amongst others), contains details of all live births, stillbirths and deaths, plus notifications of infectious diseases. These are tabled as six-week cumulative totals and as numbers for the current week. It lists newly diagnosed episodes of communicable and respiratory diseases as well as the weekly numbers and rates.

PROFESSIONAL GUIDELINES AND EDUCATION ISSUES

Many professional bodies have written guidelines on the management of communicable diseases, and the Institute of Environmental Health Officers has published an excellent manual about the acquired immune deficiency syndrome, AIDS (Institute of Environmental Health Officers, 1987, and see chapter 10). This is an explicit but easy to read booklet containing a wealth of information, practical advice and discussion on legal and ethical issues. Although not legally bound by it, professionals have a responsibility to be aware of and follow the expert advice disseminated by their institutions or professional organisations.

As far as AIDS is concerned perhaps the most active forum for producing and publicising accurate and relevant information has come from the voluntary sector, particularly The Terence Higgins Trust. This is a charity which has pioneered support services and acts as a resource centre for AIDS sufferers and those involved with them. Its many publications are aimed at a wide population and a reading list may be obtained from them at BM AIDS, London, WC1N 3XX.

Further information and a wide variety of teaching material on AIDS and other

Table 9.3 Communicable disease surveillance data collection

Active data collection
Special epidemiological surveys specifically designed for the purposes of surveillance

Passive data collection
Routine national reporting systems providing data for surveillance
- *Laboratory reporting*   The PHLS reporting system from medical microbiologists to the CDSC
- *Statutory notification*   Central reporting to OPCS of locally notified infectious disease
- *Clinical reporting from general practice*   Central collection by the Royal College of General Practitioners of clinical data from selected general practices
- *Clinical reporting from hospital specialists*   Examples are the British Paediatric Surveillance Unit for rare paediatric disorders and selected specialists for AIDS and HIV symptomatic patients
- *Morbidity data*   from the Medical Officer of Schools Association
- *Hospital data*   Central collection by the OPCS of data on hospital discharges and deaths
- *Mortality data*   Central collection by the OPCS of data from death certification and registration

(See text for abbreviations. From Galbraith, 1986. Reproduced by kind permission of *Midwife, Health Visitor and Community Nurse*.)

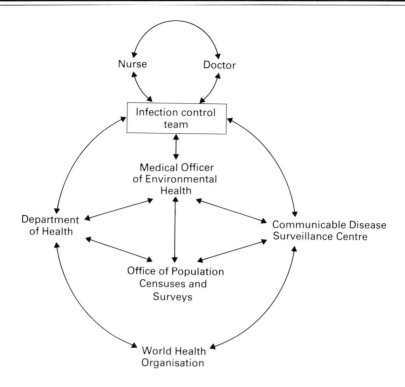

Fig 9.2 Entities involved in the monitoring and reporting of notifiable disease

infectious diseases can also be obtained from the Health Education Authority, the Royal College of Nursing and the British Medical Association.

Again, on a national basis, the Department of the Secretary of State for Health produces a quarterly report on AIDS in the form of a press release compiled from data collected by the Communicable Disease Surveillance Centre.

Hospital- and community based staff are an integral part of the national and international team responsible for the surveillance of communicable diseases (figure 9.2). Many agencies rely heavily on their observation and communication skills to achieve the WHO objective of 'health for all by the year 2000'.

References

Acheson R M and Hagard S (1984) *Health, Society and Medicine*, 3rd edn. Oxford: Blackwell Scientific Publications.

Donaldson R J and Donaldson L J (1983) *Essential Community Medicine*. Lancaster: MTP Press.

Galbraith N S (1982) Communicable disease surveillance. In: *Recent Advances in Community Medicine*, ed. Smith A, 2nd edn., p. 127. Edinburgh: Churchill Livingstone.

Galbraith N S (1986) Infectious disease control. *Midwife, Health Visitor and Community Nurse*, **22**: 230.

Galbraith N S and Young S E J (1980) Communicable disease control: the development of a laboratory associated national epidemiological service in England and Wales. *Community Medicine*, **2**: 135.

Institution of Environmental Health Officers (1987) *Acquired Immune Deficiency Syndrome: Guidance Notes for Environmental Health Officers*. London: IEHO.

Lucas A O (1974) In: *Public Health in Europe 3: Communicable Diseases*. Copenhagen: World Health Organisation.

Raska K (1969) *The Concept of Epidemiological Surveillance. Communicable Diseases: Methods of Surveillance*. Report on a seminar convened by the Regional Office for Europe of the World Health Organisation. Copenhagen: World Health Organisation.

Further Reading

Barker D J P and Rose G (1976) *Epidemiology in Medical Practice*. Edinburgh: Churchill Livingstone.

Cartwright F F (1977) *A Social History of Medicine*. London: Longman.

Creighton C (1965) *A History of Epidemics in Britain*. London: Frank Cass.

Department of Health and Social Security (1976) *Memorandum on Lassa Fever*. London: HMSO.

Galbraith N S (1985) Infectious disease and human travel. In: *Recent Advances in Community Medicine*, ed. Smith A. Edinburgh: Churchill Livingstone.

Galbraith N S and Barrett N J (1987) Changing patterns of communicable disease. *Health and Hygiene*, **8**: 102–117.

Galbraith N S, Forbes P and Mayton-White R T (1980) Changing patterns of communicable disease in England and Wales. *British Medical Journal*, **281**: 427–430, 489–492, 546–549.

Lancet Editorial (1985) Voluntary agreements do not stop epidemics. *Lancet*, **ii** 855.

Monath T P (1975) Lassa fever: review of epidemiology and epixootiology. *WHO Bulletin*, **52**: 577–592.

Taylor I, Tomlinson A J M and Davies J R (1962) Diphtheria control in the 1960s. *Royal Society of Health Journal*, **82**: 158.

Velimirovic B (1984) *Infectious Diseases in Europe*. Copenhagen: World Health Organisation.

10

Changing Patterns of

Microbial Disease

There have been many, varied factors which have changed the pattern of infectious disease over the centuries, long before the development of immunisation or antibiotics. The opening chapter of this book considered those factors; this closing chapter looks at current trends and disease patterns.

The twentieth century has brought with it many environmental improvements in the developed countries including the provision of safe water supplies, safe sewage and waste disposal systems, improved food and milk hygiene and better control of insects and pests. Better nutrition and the introduction of vaccines and antibiotics have resulted in the disappearance of some diseases, e.g. smallpox, and a marked reduction in others, such as tuberculosis, diphtheria and poliomyelitis. Better methods of surveillance, new drugs and vaccines continue to emerge, and improved health education probably reaches a wider audience than before.

INFECTIOUS DISEASE IN THE UK

Despite improvements in living conditions in general, however, potentially serious yet preventable diseases continue to occur. In the UK, there has been a big increase in the incidence of gastroenteritis, although the notification of gastrointestinal infections always represents the 'tip of the iceberg' as many food-borne illnesses go unreported or the sufferers never seek treatment (see section on Salmonella below).

Similarly, infections with salmonella and rotavirus have continued to increase during the last decade, although infection by enteropathogenic *Escherichia coli* in children under three years of age has declined.

Reported gastrointestinal infections due to campylobacter have exceeded those caused by salmonella, but this may be partly due to improved methods of detecting the organism in the stools. Some people argue that it is the method of detection that has changed the figures and not the prevalence of the organisms themselves.

In recent years, antibiotic administration itself has become the cause of an increase in the incidence of some infections, such as pseudomembranous colitis caused by *Clostridium difficile* toxin.

In the UK in 1987, methicillin-resistant *Staphylococcus aureus* (MRSA) infection and colonisation became a significant problem, especially in North London hospitals. A similar resistance had occurred in the 1950s, when the bacteriophage type 80/81 became resistant to antibiotics, transmitting this to its host bacteria, and the high level of resulting cross-infection necessitated the closure of some hospital wards. This became pandemic and, in an effort to control the situation, a new scheme of infection control was developed in one region that decided to employ the services of an infection control sister (Gardner et al, 1962).

Another disease which shows a periodic increase in incidence in England and Wales is meningococcal meningitis, an epidemic of which recently occurred in 1987.

Hepatitis B is endemic in many tropical countries and had an increasing incidence in the UK, which has decreased dramatically since 1984 (see p. 224). The first vaccine was expensive and was, therefore, only given to NHS health-care workers, such as dentists, surgeons and laboratory workers, who were at particular risk. A much cheaper vaccine was made available in 1987 which should mean that hepatitis B need no longer be an occupational hazard for health-care workers.

INFECTIOUS DISEASE FROM ABROAD

Although many infectious diseases have been either eliminated or controlled in developed countries, they continue to occur in those still developing. Examples of these are tuberculosis and salmonellosis (including typhoid fever). The rapid and continuing increase in international travel allows cases of these illnesses to appear in the UK with increasing frequency.

Typhoid fever remains mainly an imported disease, with 30 of the 33 cases notified in 1987 thought to have been contracted abroad (Communicable Disease Report, 1986). A high percentage of cases of salmonellosis and campylobacter enteritis notified in the UK also originates in other countries, despite the increasing native incidence of these illnesses.

Travel also allows the importation of infectious diseases such as Lassa fever to countries where physicians have little or no previous experience of them, which may make diagnosis slow and difficult. Although malaria is sometimes mistakenly thought to be Lassa fever, a carefully taken history will help to clarify the situation. Lassa fever is a disease endemic only in a clearly defined part of Africa and is unlikely to be contracted unless the traveller has visited rural areas.

Prophylactic human immunoglobulin against hepatitis A is recommended for those travelling to countries where the water supply may be contaminated.

Anyone wishing to travel abroad is able to consult his general practitioner about the need for immunisation and/or prophylaxis against many infections, including malaria. Information on malaria is constantly being updated as fluctuations appear in the incidence of the disease and antimalarial resistance emerges. The Medical Service for Travellers Abroad at the London School of Hygiene and Tropical Medicine will provide detailed information.

Although thorough screening of blood for transfusions has been maintained at a high standard in developed countries, measures have been sought by some who fear they risk acquiring HIV or other viral infections should they need blood transfusions while abroad. As a result, some insurance companies, for an increased premium, offer immediate air transport to a UK hospital in an emergency.

'NEW' INFECTIOUS ILLNESSES

As well as infections being imported in increasing frequency, so-called 'new diseases' have arisen in recent years. Legionnaires' disease, caused by a bacterium commonly found in water, is certainly not new but has found a new way of transmitting infection via air-conditioning systems. This disease is a common cause of concern, both for holiday-makers abroad and for those working in large, air-conditioned buildings in the UK.

Acquired immune deficiency syndrome (AIDS) caused by the human immunodeficiency virus (HIV) is the most recently identified and serious communicable disease. The number of reports of AIDS cases has continued to double every 10 or 11 months since it was first described, and there has been no evidence of its levelling off. As a result of the widespread publicity and increase in health education to help prevent this disease, there has been a significant decrease in the incidence of all venereal diseases.

The organisms considered above will now be studied in more detail.

CAMPYLOBACTER

The name campylobacter, from the Greek meaning 'curved rod', was suggested by Sebald and Veron (1963) to distinguish the organism from vibrios which are part of the same family. When it was first reported at the turn of the century, it was mistaken for a spirochaete (Doenges, 1939).

Campylobacter organisms are highly motile, spiral-shaped, Gram-negative bacilli that fail to grow in air and require an atmosphere of reduced oxygen. A single flagellum is situated at one or both poles of the organism, which exhibits an extremely rapid darting motility. The principal species is *C. jejuni.*

Incidence

Campylobacter jejuni causes between 3 and 11 per cent of cases of diarrhoea worldwide and is also widespread in animals. It occurs equally in men and women, but is more common in young adults and children who are generally less affected by the disease than are adults. Close contacts are sometimes found to be symptomless carriers.

Since the 1970s when a filtering technique was developed (Butzler et al, 1973) and an antibiotic-selective agar introduced (Skirrow, 1977), there has been a continuing rise in the reported rate of its isolation (figure 10.1). Previously, recovery of the organism from stools was unsuccessful and only those which could be isolated from blood were reported.

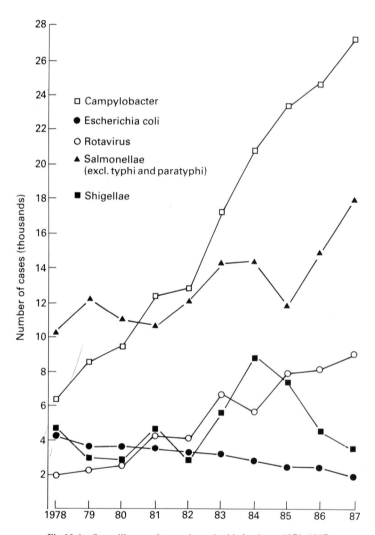

Fig 10.1 Surveillance of gastrointestinal infections, 1978–1987
(Reproduced by kind permission of the Communicable Disease Surveillance Centre)

Mode of Spread

The organism is less infectious than others causing gastroenteritis and person-to-person transmission is very uncommon, although cross-infection has been reported in households during the acute diarrhoeal phase. This person-to-person spread is usually between children but it may extend to adults handling excreta of the infected child. Vertical transmission, that is through the placenta to the foetus, does occur.

The organism is most commonly found in unpasteurised milk or cream and in chickens, both deep-frozen and freshly refrigerated. Contamination is mainly on the outer surface of the birds. A wide range of birds, wild animals and farm animals, as well as domestic pets, has been found to be carriers. Spread from handling domestic pets and other animals suffering from diarrhoea occurs more commonly. Cats and puppies are a particular risk to small children (Svedhem, 1980).

An unchlorinated public water supply was reported as the source of over 2000 cases of gastroenteritis in Vermont, USA, which had a population of only 10 000 (Tiehan and Vogt, 1978).

Incubation Period

This is about five days but ranges from two to 11 days.

Symptoms

Apart from diarrhoea, abdominal pain and cramps are the most outstanding symptoms and often persist after the diarrhoea eases. Diarrhoea may be accompanied by malaise, headache, backache, aching limbs, nausea and vomiting.

The profuse diarrhoea, which may start gradually in some and explosively in others, may last for between five and 10 days. There may also be a low-grade fever for two or three days, which is sometimes followed by rigor. Although campylobacter is infrequently isolated from the blood, obtaining it in culture from this site suggests bacteraemia or septicaemia.

In severe cases, dehydration and electrolyte disturbances may occur, with blood, pus and/or bile appearing in the offensive stools. On average the illness lasts for between 10 and 14 days. Some patients have been known to carry the organisms for months, but it is usual to obtain a negative culture in a few weeks. The low incidence of carriage in the population would suggest that the period of excretion is short.

Prevention

Essential for preventing this disease are adequate chlorination of drinking water, good husbandry by cattle and poultry farmers and safe practice in food-processing plants.

Although campylobacter commonly causes milk-borne outbreaks it is readily eliminated by pasteurisation. The practice of drinking unpasteurised milk and cream should be discouraged.

There is a need for education of the general public as well as of food handlers in the safe preparation and cooking of deep-frozen poultry. Similarly, veterinary surgeons could help by educating pet owners in the correct handling of their pets.

Since this is not a disease easily transmitted from person to person, it is unnecessary to obtain bacteriological clearance to return to work even for food handlers who should, of course, be excluded from work during the diarrhoeal phase.

Treatment

The majority of patients have a self-limiting condition requiring only treatment of the symptoms. Hospitalisation is, therefore, rarely necessary.

Campylobacter is sensitive to erythromycin and the aminoglycoside group of antibiotics. Oral erythromycin stearate (Erythrocin) has a narrow spectrum of activity, is acid-resistant and is incompletely absorbed. This gives it the advantage of exerting its effect on the lumen of the bowel and the blood. It may alleviate severe stomach cramps with profuse diarrhoea if given within two days. Gentamicin is the drug of choice when the patient is septicaemic.

It appears that campylobacter is an important cause of enteritis, the number of reported cases continuing to rise since improved methods of isolation have been developed. Serotyping, biotyping and plasmid analysis may provide useful information during an epidemic.

Since the late 1970s, there has been evidence to show that *C. pyloridis* may be associated with gastritis and peptic ulcer disease (Waghorn, 1987).

SALMONELLA

Salmonellae are pathogens of both humans and animals. They are Gram-negative organisms which are actively motile, and are one of the many groups of organisms that can cause food poisoning (Shanson, 1982). They may also cause a slowly developing persistent enteritis, typhoid or septicaemia. The latter may lead to osteomyelitis, endocarditis, pneumonia, pulmonary abscess or meningitis.

There are three recognised species:

1. *Salm. enteritidis* which includes the most commonly occurring strains, *Salm. typhimurium* (in poultry) and *Salm. dublin* (in meat). These can cause gastroenteritis within hours of ingesting contaminated food.
2. *Salm. typhi* (which causes typhoid fever) and the associated *Salm. paratyphi*.
3. *Salm. choleraesuis* which is mainly associated with the pig family and is more common in the USA than in the UK.

There are over 1700 salmonella serotypes and many are given the names of the places in which they were first isolated, e.g. Dublin and Singapore.

Incidence

Although the incidence of salmonellosis remains static in the animal population, it continues to increase in humans (see figure 10.1), being mainly acquired from poultry, both deep-frozen and freshly refrigerated. It may also be present in eggs and egg products. Salmonellae are also very common parasites of domestic, farmyard and wild animals. Salmonellosis in cattle is a bi-phasic disease coinciding with calving in the spring and autumn. There was a big increase in the incidence of the disease in the 1960s, probably due to rapid movement of stock through the country when replacements were produced for the many cattle which were destroyed with foot and mouth disease.

In the UK, the incidence of bacterial food poisoning continues to rise (Communicable Diseases Report, 1986). One contributing factor is the increasing number of people who eat in hotels and restaurants or consume 'take-away' food. At home, not defrosting poultry adequately before cooking is the most common cause of salmonella food-poisoning.

In 1980 the Public Health Laboratory Service Salmonella Subcommittee reviewed 552 hospital salmonella outbreaks in England and Wales from 1968 to 1977 (Abbot et al, 1980). Of 76 outbreaks where a source of infection was reported, food was implicated in only 24 (30 per cent). Fifty-one per cent of non-food-borne outbreaks occurred in maternity, paediatric and geriatric units compared with only 22 per cent of food-borne outbreaks.

During the Bank Holiday of August 1984 at the Stanley Royd Hospital, Wakefield, Yorkshire, an outbreak of salmonella food-poisoning began which resulted in 19 deaths. An enquiry was set up by the Secretary of State for Social Services to investigate the source of the outbreak of food poisoning, to report and to make recommendations to prevent a recurrence (Department of Health and Social Security, 1986).

Mode of Spread

Although most salmonella infections are acquired by eating or drinking contaminated items, person-to-person spread has occurred in large institutions. Since the route of transmission of salmonella is faeco-oral, person-to-person spread should not be expected in general hospitals if a high standard of hygiene can be ensured.

Typhoid fever rarely spreads from one person to another but paratyphoid occasionally does so, especially when causing a diarrhoeal illness. Its usual mode of spread is through contaminated food or sewage-polluted water.

Symptoms

The symptoms of salmonellosis are contained in table 10.1.

Table 10.1 Symptoms of salmonellosis

Organism	Incubation period	Predominating symptoms	Duration of illness
Salm. enteritidis (*Salm. typhimurium and others*)	8–48 hours	Nausea, vomiting, diarrhoea, fever	1–4 days
Salm. typhi, *Salm. paratyphi*	7–20 days	Fever, abdominal tenderness, rash, prostration, bacteraemia	1–3 weeks
All serotypes but mainly *Salm. choleraesuis*	Variable	Spiking fever, septicaemia	Weeks to months
All serotypes	Variable	Localised infection, abscess formation	Weeks

Prevention

Pre-employment screening for salmonella is not recommended for any occupation and routine screening of catering staff is inappropriate (Public Health Laboratory Service Salmonella Sub-Committee, 1983). It must be stressed to all food handlers that they must never work if they are suffering from diarrhoea and that they must submit a stool specimen for examination. Once the stools are normal and well-formed, the employee may return to work.

Outbreaks of salmonellosis are preventable provided that all staff maintain good personal hygiene and that the basic rules for storage, preparation, cooking and serving of food are obeyed. A continuing education programme should be available to all food handlers in all establishments and institutions.

Salmonellae can survive drying and cold temperatures (such as refrigeration), but are easily destroyed by pasteurisation. Separation of cooked and raw meat during storage and preparation is essential to prevent contamination.

The Committee of Enquiry following the Stanley Royd Hospital outbreak (see above) made a number of preventive recommendations mainly related to improving poor facilities and practices in the kitchens. In addition, it recommended a reduction in the number of elderly senile mentally ill (ESMI) patients housed together, and emphasised the need for adequate numbers of appropriately trained staff, particularly nurses.

In 1987 Crown Immunity was removed from UK hospitals, and one of the results has been that health authorities whose catering departments do not comply with requirements are liable to prosecution.

Although salmonellae are commonly found in pests, such as mice and cockroaches, in hospitals and other establishments, these have not been proven sources of outbreaks of gastroenteritis.

Treatment

Treatment by antibiotics is not routinely recommended as this may increase the period of carriage and result in an increase in the number of resistant strains. If, however, symptoms are severe or bacteraemia occurs, treatment will be required.

A carrier state can occur and may be identified in some individuals where prior disease, or exposure to it, was not suspected.

Correction of fluid and electrolyte imbalance is needed. The old and very young can quickly become dehydrated.

From the 1950s onwards, chloramphenicol was the antibiotic of choice against salmonella but, when its agranulocytic effect on bone marrow was discovered, its use was restricted to cases of typhoid only. Unfortunately, in some countries it is available over the chemist's counter and, in 1972 in Mexico, its indiscriminate use resulted in more than 10 000 cases of typhoid fever resistant to chloramphenicol (Baldry, 1976).

CLOSTRIDIUM DIFFICILE

Clostridium difficile is a Gram-positive, sporing bacillus which produces two toxins: an enterotoxin and a cytotoxin. The spores can survive for long periods, probably for months, in the inanimate environment. The bacterium's pathogenicity was not recognised until its cytotoxin was implicated as the cause of pseudomembranous colitis, first with the results of a study by Larson et al in 1977. They showed a previously unidentified toxin in the faeces of patients who developed pseudomembranous colitis after treatment with penicillin.

Incidence

Clostridium difficile is commonly recovered from the stools of infants but seldom from those of healthy adults. It has been reported in 35 per cent of neonates admitted to a neonatal intensive care unit (Donta and Myers, 1982), and up to 56 per cent of adults with antibiotic-associated diarrhoea. It has also been cultured from the vagina of many asymptomatic women.

Normal faecal flora may suppress *Cl. difficile*, so that patients undergoing antibiotic therapy which destroys the normal flora may be at greatest risk of acquiring the organism and developing colitis. Most cases reported have followed treatment with ampicillin, clindamycin or a cephalosporin but other antibiotics have also been implicated.

Hafiz et al (1975) isolated the bacterium more often from the urogenital tracts of patients attending 'special' (venereology) clinics than from those of their control subjects. It was found in 72 per cent of 108 women and 100 per cent of 42 men with non-specific urethritis. In a study of elderly hospital in-patients, *Cl. difficile* was found in two thirds of those admitted suffering from diarrhoea (Treloar and Kalra, 1987). These results suggest that *Cl. difficile* plays an important part in causing diarrhoeal infections.

Mode of Spread

Clostridium difficile toxins are the most important cause of antibiotic-associated colitis, but the sources of the organism and its method of transmission are still incompletely defined.

Colitis has been recognised as a complication of antimicrobial therapy since the 1950s. It is unclear whether it is the result of overgrowth of *Cl. difficile* in a symptomless carrier, or whether it is acquired from other patients or from the environment. Some hospital outbreaks have been reported which could suggest exogenous infection, and it is possible that the organism may survive in spore form for months in the environment.

Kim et al (1981) showed that the prevalence of *Cl. difficile* was significantly higher in areas where there were known cases of antibiotic-associated diarrhoea, and a higher rate of positive culture was obtained when diarrhoeal symptoms were present than when they were not. Results, however, were not sufficient to incriminate the environment, and both food and air sampling proved negative.

Symptoms

Profuse, watery diarrhoea becoming progressively more severe may be accompanied by fever, vomiting, abdominal cramps or peritonitis. Acute inflammation of the large bowel develops and an apparent membrane covers the damaged mucosa. This 'pseudomembrane' is made up of plaques of exudate.

Prevention

Prevention of the disease not only involves the control of the antibiotics which precipitate it, but also demands the clarification of the potential chain of transmission between healthy people, animals and the environment.

Although environmental contamination occurs readily during outbreaks when there is incontinence, transmission is preventable provided that staff wash and dry their hands thoroughly between attending different patients. Wearing disposable gloves and aprons when attending such incontinent patients may help to reduce the risk of transmission. Nursing in a single room is also advisable where one is available.

Since *Cl. difficile* is a spore-producing organism, the cleaning and disinfection of sigmoidoscopes, colonoscopes etc. needs to be thorough. An agent which will ensure that spores are destroyed must be used, e.g. 2 per cent gluteraldehyde for 30 minutes.

Treatment

The most effective treatment for pseudomembranous colitis is oral vancomycin, 125–500 mg six-hourly. This produces rapid alleviation of symptoms and eradication of *Cl. difficile* and its toxins (Keighley et al, 1978).

Metronidazole is well absorbed from the gut and there have been reports that a 10-day oral course of 400 mg t.d.s can be effective (Bolton, 1980). Symptoms may resolve with antidiarrhoeal agents alone (Kappas et al, 1978).

Recurrences do occur and may be a consequence of the failure to eradicate the spores from the intestine.

Despite recently-developed methods for typing *Cl. difficile*, the major means of spread remains unclear. Although it can be recovered from the environment for some time after it has been eradicated from the patient's stools, there is currently insufficient evidence specifically to incriminate the surroundings.

LEGIONNAIRES' DISEASE

Legionella pneumophila was identified in January 1977 as the organism which had caused so-called Legionnaires' disease in Philadelphia, USA, the previous year among delegates at an American Legion conference. Since then, 22 legionella species have been identified. Legionella is a water-borne agent which has caused outbreaks of disease in hospitals and hotels, mainly by colonising the cooling towers of air-conditioning systems (Helms et al, 1983).

Incidence

The incidence of Legionnaire's disease is higher in men than women, and attack rates increase progressively with age. The risk of acquiring the disease appears higher in smokers and those who have other respiratory diseases or who suffer from diabetes, cancer or renal disease.

During 1987, 10 cases of Legionnaires' disease were reported among British visitors returning from Yugoslavia, and from the Netherlands one case was confirmed and four suspected. Five cases were reported from a hotel in Portugal where two cases had been reported earlier in the year. Seven were reported from Spain; two of the victims stayed in the same hotel and the other five stayed at hotels which had been associated with cases the previous year (Communicable Disease Report, 1987b).

In May 1988, a cooling tower at the BBC's Broadcasting House in London was suspected of causing an outbreak of Legionnaires' disease and was taken out of operation. One month later, 26 cases were confirmed and a further 45 suspected. All of the victims had visited or worked within 500 m of the building, although several had only briefly visited the area and probably contracted the disease while walking in the street outside (Communicable Disease Report, 1988a). Investigation of patients admitted to hospital with pneumonia is advised during outbreaks of this kind.

Mode of Spread

Human-to-human transmission has not been reported and, therefore, reliance is on prevention of the infection by correct maintenance of plumbing and air-conditioning systems.

Symptoms

Legionnaires' disease is a systemic bacterial infection, manifested particularly as pneumonia. Symptoms can vary from a mild influenza-like illness to a fulminant pneumonia. Extra-pulmonary infection has also been reported in the form of prosthetic valve endocarditis, wound infections, sinusitis, peritonitis, pericarditis and abscesses of other organs (Edelstein, 1986).

Prevention

Prevention aims to eliminate or reduce the presence of *Legionella pneumophila* to the absolute minimum in institutions, hospitals and hotels. To achieve this, knowledge of the factors promoting colonisation and growth are necessary. Water stagnation, hot water storage tanks and plumbing dead-ends can all help to promote growth and should be avoided.

Regardless of which method of disinfection is used it is often difficult to eliminate legionella completely. The presence of algae facilitates the multiplication of legionella; therefore, regular cleaning and descaling of cooling towers and water tanks acts as a deterrent.

In hospitals a planned, preventive maintenance programme, carried out by the engineering department, is essential. Correct chlorination of the water supply and elevation of hot water temperatures have proved effective control measures (Fisher Hoch et al, 1981); indeed, the two most successful methods of disinfection for ending outbreaks have been chlorination and pasteurisation. The method used includes continuous heating of the water to 60°C, combined with chlorination of the incoming water. This regime can prove expensive for hospitals, and it is also important to warn staff and patients of the danger of scalding from the hot water.

Department of Health and Social Security guidelines relating to the management of cooling towers and evaporating condensers were issued to all health authorities in May 1987 (Department of Health and Social Security, 1987a). The DHSS also published recommendations on the use of hot and cold water distribution systems (Department of Health and Social Security, 1987b).

Treatment

Erythromycin and rifampicin are the recognised antibiotics for treating Legionnaire's disease. They should be given for several weeks as relapses have been reported when the drugs have been prescribed for only a fortnight. Cotrimoxazole and tetracycline are sometimes used. Beta-lactam and aminoglycoside antibiotics are ineffective.

METHICILLIN-RESISTANT STAPHYLOCOCCUS AUREUS

Staphylococcus aureus remains a major cause of surgical sepsis and septicaemia despite the introduction of antibiotics (see chapters 2 and 7).

Incidence

In the 1950s, a virulent strain of *Staph. aureus* became resistant to penicillin, streptomycin, tetracycline, erythromycin and novobiocin. No explanation has been found for the gradual decline of this organism which then occurred during the 1960s. Methicillin was introduced in the 1960s, and hopes were raised that it would combat the problem of penicillin resistance. Unfortunately, by 1976, a strain which was resistant to both gentamicin and methicillin was first reported in Britain, as well as increasingly causing outbreaks in the USA, Australia and Eire. Epidemics of methicillin-resistant *Staph. aureus* (MRSA) infection have been increasingly reported in Britain since 1980 (Price, 1984; Selkon et al, 1980), although many of the patients were colonised rather than infected.

Moderately severe infections involving soft tissues, bones and joints, postoperative wounds, urinary tracts and lungs have been reported. More serious infections in patients who have indwelling intravenous catheters or prosthetic heart valves may result in death from septicaemia and endocarditis.

Experience of recent outbreaks suggests that the main risk of serious MRSA infection occurs in patients in special units, e.g. ITU, cardiothoracic and surgical neonatal units, and in patients undergoing major or prosthetic surgery. The elderly are especially likely to become colonised and act as a source of infection, particularly when admitted to acute surgical units.

A particular strain which has caused a number of outbreaks in the Thames health region has been given the name epidemic MRSA (EMRSA) (Cook and Marples, 1985). At present it remains sensitive to vancomycin, which is expensive and requires frequent serum drug concentration checks to prevent toxic side-effects.

Mode of Spread

The most important mode of spread for MRSA is, probably, contact transmission by the hands of hospital personnel. There is no evidence for contact transmission by fomites (i.e. inanimate objects). Cultures taken from the environment have generally proved negative during outbreaks except in burns units (Crossley et al, 1979; Rutala et al, 1983).

The most consistent finding when looking at risk factors for the acquisition of MRSA is previous antibiotic therapy, particularly with penicillin, cephalosporins or aminoglycosides. One study identified, in addition, advanced age and a high number of invasive procedures as risk factors (Ward et al, 1981).

It has been demonstrated that the carrier state is far less important than the person's ability to disperse the organisms in the air. Shedding occurs in 10 per cent of male carriers and only 1 per cent of female carriers. Men also disperse organisms in greater numbers (White, 1961).

Prevention

Rapid identification and source isolation of those infected or colonised with MRSA is recommended. Precautions include the wearing of disposable gloves and aprons for contact with body fluids or changing wound dressings. Strict attention to hand-washing is of paramount importance.

Since airborne transmission has not been established for MRSA, even in burns units where MRSA may be recovered from the air, the main mode of transmission appears to be direct contact. Cohort nursing can play a very important part in minimising spread. This proposes that a patient suffering from MRSA infection or colonisation is cared for in one area of the ward, with hospital personnel assigned to work only with him. Clear, written instructions outlining necessary precautions must accompany the patient who is transferred to another hospital or institution, or who leaves hospital to be cared for by community nurses.

Cookson et al (1987) reported a marked reduction in the incidence of MRSA by employing strict isolation of patients or cohort nursing, and using chlorhexidine/alcohol hand-rub. Screening of staff and contacts and decontamination with mupirocin were also employed (Cookson et al, 1987).

Infections are reported from all common sites. Except for blood or intra-abdominal abscesses which can only be infected, other sites may be either colonised or infected; in all instances they are an important reservoir of MRSA which they may harbour for many months. Since patients tend to remain colonised for many months they should, ideally, be routinely isolated if they are readmitted to hospital for screening. Some indication to this effect needs to be made on the patient's notes, and close liaison should be maintained between the community and hospital nursing services.

The control of outbreaks has proved difficult and, once it has been introduced into a hospital, many have been unable to totally eradicate MRSA from in-patients, particularly where there are smouldering reservoirs such as decubitus ulcers. If every effort is made to prevent pressure sores and heal varicose ulcers, the incidence of MRSA colonisation in care of the elderly hospitals would probably be reduced.

Some argue that it is difficult to prove that screening of all staff and other patients in the ward during an outbreak justifies the expense involved. Staff who carry MRSA have not been proved to be an important reservoir unless found also to be dispersers of staphylococcus.

Treatment

Eradication of MRSA has proved to be extremely difficult and, where successful, is often only temporary. Locksley et al (1982) reported success by using intravenous vancomycin and oral rifampicin, but three out of eight patients relapsed one to three weeks after completing therapy.

Variable results have been reported from those attempting eradication of the organism using topical antimicrobials, including lysostaphin, gentamicin, neomycin, chlorhexidine, vancomycin and bacitracin. Others have been equally unsuccessful in eradicating the carrier state.

MENINGOCOCCAL MENINGITIS

The most common groups of meningococcus are A, B, C, D, X, Y, Z, E29 and W135. It is an aerobic, non-motile organism for which only humans are the natural host.

Incidence

In the UK, meningococcal meningitis is a notifiable disease and local health officials must be notified of each case. Records from all over England and Wales are kept at the Communicable Disease Surveillance Centre (CDSC) in London. The picture changes from year to year. There was a peak of 12 000 cases in a single year at the time of the Second World War. In the mid 1970s, there was a rise to between 1100 and 1200 cases, and the incidence is again rising, with a figure of 1331 for 1987 which is double that of the early 1980s (figure 10.2). The 1970s outbreak was caused entirely by group B strains and the current rise includes groups B and C. Group A organisms seem to have been fairly insignificant throughout, and relatively rare in the UK.

In the UK from October 1981–86 there were 98 cases of meningococcal disease reported by Gloucester Health Authority, which has a population of 300 000. An expected figure would be 30 (Cartwright et al, 1986; Cartwright, 1987). The outbreak was carefully monitored by the Public Health Laboratory Service, and the distribution of the strains and the prevalence of immunity to them was studied. It was found that there was a low carriage rate of the strains causing the outbreak in the community in which the disease was active. This supports the theory that the 'outbreak' meningococci are more virulent but less transmissible than other strains

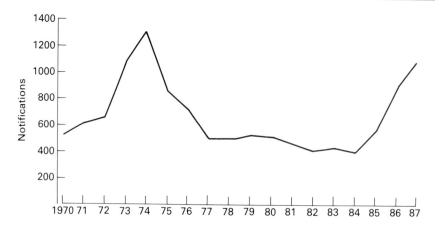

Fig 10.2　Annual notifications of meningococcal meningitis in England and Wales, 1970–1987 (Reproduced by kind permission of the Communicable Disease Surveillance Centre)

of meningococci. Up to the 49th week of 1987, 1036 notifications of meningococcal meningitis were received by the CDSC in London. These show an increase in the number of group C infections and a fall in those caused by group B organisms (Communicable Disease Report, 1987d).

Although 21 cases of acute group A meningoccal infection have been identified in England, the sufferers had all returned from Mecca or were domestic contacts of pilgrims returning from Mecca (Communicable Disease Report, 1987a). As a result, vaccination is advised for anyone likely to spend more than a few days in certain countries.

Mode of Spread

The only important source of this organism, *Neisseria meningitidis*, is the nasopharynx either of patients with clinical disease or of asymptomatic carriers. It is spread only by close, direct contact and dies rapidly on exposure to the environment.

Symptoms

During the nasopharyngeal colonisation stage, there may be a mild respiratory illness. The organism may enter the central lymph nodes and thus reach the bloodstream. It can then spread through the body, leading to a petechial skin rash and also causing petechial lesions in the joints, heart and lungs.

The signs of meningeal irritation become apparent with stiff neck, retraction of the head and a positive Kernig's sign i.e. the inability to straighten the knee joint when the hip joint is flexed. In severe cases, there may be opisthotonos.

Between 20 and 40 per cent of cases of meningitis occur without overt signs of bacteriaemia. Where meningococcaemia does occur, it may cause acute symptoms and can be fatal within 12 hours.

Prevention

Source isolation precautions are only required for the first 48 hours after the start of appropriate antibiotic therapy. A single room is preferable as the patient often suffers from photophobia and needs to be in a darkened room away from noise and light.

Chemoprophylaxis is necessary for close contacts only (i.e. the family). Prophylaxis is recommended for health-care workers only if mouth-to-mouth resuscitation has been necessary before the patient had received antibiotic therapy (Communicable Disease Report, 1981).

Meningococcal polysaccharide vaccine (against strains A and C) is available on a named-patient basis. This may be useful in the control of outbreaks of these specific groups. Side-effects have been reported more commonly in children under two years of age. These are usually febrile reactions.

Rifampicin is the agent recommended for treating close contacts to remove possible nasopharyngeal carriage. The drug is contraindicated in pregnancy as there is a risk of teratogenicity. It is also necessary to warn patients that rifampicin can cause orange discolouration of urine and tears, stain contact lenses and affect the action of the contraceptive pill.

Treatment

Two mega units of benzylpenicillin are given intravenously two-hourly for the first 24–48 hours. This is followed for a minimum of 10 to 14 days by 2 mega units four-hourly.

For penicillin-allergic patients, chloramphenicol is given, 1 g q.d.s. intravenously for the first 48 hours, followed by the same dose orally for between 10 and 14 days.

Some of the second or third generation cephalosporins may become future alternatives to these drugs.

ACQUIRED IMMUNE DEFICIENCY SYNDROME

Acquired immune deficiency syndrome (AIDS) is caused by the human immuno-deficiency virus (HIV), a retrovirus which attacks and destroys the T helper cells in the blood stream (see chapter 3). Since these T helper cells stimulate cellular immunity in the presence of antigen, the body's ability to destroy invading microorganisms becomes much reduced. All microorganisms, including fungi, protozoa and even the patient's own flora, become potentially pathogenic.

The virus replicates within the living cells from which it is able to bud out and infect more of the host's cells. The sufferer's blood is infectious once antibodies are detectable, but it is not yet clear when this state gives rise to illness in the host.

Terms commonly encountered when considering AIDS and HIV are:

- *ARC* AIDS-related complex
- *PGL* Persistent generalised lymphadenopathy
- *PCP* *Pneumocystis carinii* pneumonia
- *AZT* Azidothymidine (Zidovudine), an antiviral agent

Incidence

The cumulative totals of UK reports of AIDS up to April 1988 show 1417 cases in men, with 812 deaths, and 46 cases in women, with 27 deaths (table 10.2). Of the men, 88 per cent were homosexual or bisexual (Communicable Disease Report, 1988b).

Mode of Spread

HIV has been isolated from many body fluids. Transmission, however, has been definitely associated only with semen, blood and blood products. There are three methods of transmission recognised:

1. Injection or transfusion of blood or blood products from an infected person
2. Sexual contact (from virus present in the semen)
3. Intrauterine or perinatally from mother to baby

The high incidence of HIV among homosexual men is partly due to the high number of sexual contacts involved, but is also due to anal intercourse where semen

Table 10.2 UK AIDS cases by patient characteristics: cumulative totals to end September 1988

	Males	Females	Total	Deaths
Homosexual/bisexual	1475	–	1475	790
Intravenous drug abuser	26	10	36	20
Homosexual and intravenous drug abuser	29	–	29	14
Haemophiliac	117	1	118	73
Recipient of blood:				
Abroad	10	10	20	13
UK	9	3	12	10
Heterosexual:				
Presumed infected abroad	38	17	55	20
Presumed infected UK	5	7	12	8
Child of at-risk or infected parent	8	11	19	7
Other undetermined	16	2	19	10
Totals	1733	61	1794	965

Table prepared from voluntary confidential reports by clinicians sent directly to the PHLS Communicable Disease Surveillance Centre (01-200 6868) and to the Communicable Diseases (Scotland) Unit (041-946 7120). From *The Lancet*, 22 October 1988, reproduced by kind permission of the Communicable Disease Surveillance Centre.

is in contact with the mucosal surface of the rectum. The mucosa can be traumatised and may bleed during anal intercourse, which greatly increases the risk of transmission of the virus.

Adler (1986) estimated that between 10 and 15 per cent of homosexual men also engage in heterosexual intercourse, potentially putting their female partners at risk. Whether women are able to pass infection to men is uncertain, as there is insufficient data related to this. HIV has been isolated from the cervical and vaginal secretions of antibody positive females but the methodology of studies to prove its transmission have, to date, made the resulting evidence unreliable.

Some men and women engage in prostitution in order to support their need for illicit drugs and, as intravenous drug abusers, they are already at great risk of acquiring HIV from sharing contaminated equipment such as needles.

About one third of the 7600 haemophiliacs in the UK have antibodies to HIV. This is mainly due to the contamination of their blood factor VIII treatment made in the USA (Wells, 1986). The heat treatment now applied to blood products and the screening of donated blood should ensure that further instances of infection in this group are rare.

Advice regarding the test for HIV antibodies can be obtained from general practitioners, genitourinary medicine clinics, helplines, etc., but it is only given after counselling by a properly trained person. It is essential that the client understands the significance of a positive HIV test and the necessity for repeating the test should it be negative while he or she remains in an 'at risk' situation.

The proportion of antibody positive subjects progressing to AIDS lies between 20 and 30 per cent according to current statistics (Miller et al, 1986). New tests for serological monitoring continue to emerge. Positive HIV culture is still the only technique for demonstrating the intact virus but core antigen (p24) can be detected in the blood. Increase in the blood p24 level may indicate an increase in viral replication and enables evaluation of the effectiveness of antiviral chemotherapy. The ability to detect antigenaemia before the production of antibody offers a method of earlier detection of HIV-infected individuals. A decrease in anti-p24 and the appearance of antigen can be highly predictive of progression to AIDS. Presence of the antigen in cerebrospinal fluid has a direct relationship with progressive encephalopathy (Lombardo, 1988).

Symptoms

Opportunistic infections or tumour are the usual presenting symptom and confirm the diagnosis of AIDS. During the phase when antibodies are being produced there may be transient non-specific illnesses which include malaise, myalgia, lymphadenopathy, pharyngitis and a rash.

The chronic phase may or may not be symptomatic. According to Pinching (1986) the symptoms can be divided into two principle groups: persistent generalised lymphadenopathy (PGL) and AIDS-related complex (ARC). He maintains that those in the first group remain well whereas those in the second group suffer systemic symptoms such as weight loss, fever and diarrhoea.

Despite the progressive deterioration of the immune system, many of the infections may be treated successfully in the early stages of the disease. However the patient may need to attend hospital more and more frequently as time passes.

The vascular tumour Kaposi's sarcoma does not occur in all cases of AIDS but, in some, it may be the presenting symptom. The lesions may be small, petechial and purplish in colour, or may initially be thought to be unresolved bruising. Some lesions may be more heavily pigmented and nodular. They can occur anywhere on the skin or mucous membranes and can spread to the lymphatic system, gastrointestinal tract and other internal organs.

There can be cerebral involvement as a result of HIV infection which can present in different ways. In the early stages, this is only detected by sophisticated neuropsychometric testing but, later, memory loss and concentration problems appear. These can become confused with the more common neurological effects of opportunistic infections of the central nervous system, e.g. cryptococcal meningitis or cerebral abscess. HIV encephalopathy or AIDS-related dementia is usually a feature of late disease, but there has been a small number of patients who develop encephalopathy before developing the signs of immunosuppression.

Children infected with HIV, particularly those congenitally affected, have a poor prognosis. They are rarely asymptomatic after two years of age and approximately 50 per cent die after three years. The most common causes of death are opportunistic infection and severe encephalopathy.

The psychological problem which the HIV-positive person has to face are monumental. He or she faces the knowledge that an incurable disease may be developing, that it is communicable to others with the same possible outcome or, much worse, that the sufferer may already have transmitted it to the one person who is most important to them. Male homosexuals may have previously kept their sexual orientation a secret from their friends and relatives. Sufferers are most frequently in the age group where they are seeking insurance policies and mortgages and, should they reveal that they are HIV-seropositive, they run the risk of rejection by the majority of companies.

Initially, there is often fear and denial of the diagnosis, but this is usually followed by feelings of anger and then depression before, in many cases, coming to terms with the condition (Allen and Mellin, 1982).

Prevention

There is, as yet, no vaccine available, so efforts at curtailing the spread of the disease must be concentrated on educating the public on how it is spread and how it may be avoided.

Homosexuals are advised to adopt safer sexual practices and to reduce the number of their sexual contacts. The use of condoms is advocated for both homosexuals and heterosexuals unless they are certain that they and their partner have a monogamous sexual relationship.

The risk of health-care workers acquiring the disease through their occupation is very low. Where they are likely to come into contact with infected blood, cuts and lesions of the hands need to be covered. Care must also be taken to prevent splash of blood into the eyes or mouth. Guidelines for nursing AIDS patients have been published by the Royal College of Nursing (Royal College of Nursing, 1987a).

Clear guidelines are given by the British Dental Association (BDA) for the control of cross-infection in routine dental practice (British Dental Association, 1987). They recommend that the only safe approach is to assume that any patient may be a carrier of HIV. It is, therefore, necessary to strike a balance between cumbersome 'perfect' procedures and a reasonable approach, which is practical while minimising the hazards to a point where they present a negligible risk.

Spillages of infected blood can be safely removed using bleach or hypochlorite 1 per cent, a disposable cloth and disposable gloves. There are a number of powdered chemical products now available which release chlorine on contact with fluid spillage, so enabling safer and easier disposal.

It is unnecessary to isolate the patient on admission to hospital although he or she or the other patients may prefer it; each person needs individual assessment. It is unnecessary for those attending the patient to wear protective clothing except disposable gloves and an apron when handling blood or blood contaminated fluids. Although some would prefer that gloves are worn in contact with all body fluids this can be distressing for a patient who may already feel that he is being treated as lepers once were.

The avoidance of needlestick injuries should be stressed. Studies of transmission routes and the amount of associated infection risk, evaluated in over 3500 medical and dental workers with intensive occupational exposure to HIV, indicate an infection rate of 0.1 per cent per year of exposure (Geberding and Henderson, 1987).

There are numerous reliable sources of information for all groups of people regarding the prevention of HIV. Also, there are many telephone helplines in addition to the original, the Terence Higgins Trust. Most sexually transmissable disease clinics have a 'walk-in' advice service available as well as their regular appointment system facilities.

Treatment

There is, as yet, no treatment which will destroy HIV, but the associated life-threatening opportunistic infections need to be treated to prolong life and improve its quality. Treatment should be a three-pronged attack: prompt recognition and treatment of opportunistic infections, followed by prophylaxis against or suppression of the microorganisms (see AZT below) and then regeneration of the immune system.

The most common of the opportunistic infections are *Pneumocystis carinii* pneumonia and gastrointestinal candidiasis (see table 10.3). In some instances, pneumonia caused by other organisms may occur, e.g. from *Mycobacterium avium intracellulare*.

Table 10.3 Common opportunistic infections affecting AIDS patients

Organism	Illness
Protozoan	
Cryptosporidium	Diarrhoea
Pneumocystis carinii	Pneumonia
Toxoplasma gondii	Pneumonia or CNS infection
Fungus	
Cryptococcus	Pulmonary, disseminated or CNS infection
Candida albicans	Oesophageal or bronchopulmonary candidiasis
Bacteria	
Mycobacterium avium intracellulare (frequently resistant to isoniazid and rifampicin)	Pulmonary or disseminated disease
Shigella	Diarrhoea
Salmonella	Diarrhoea
Campylobacter	Diarrhoea
Virus	
Herpes simplex	Mucocutaneous lesions at upper and lower ends of gastronintestinal tract
Herpes zoster	Shingles
Cytomegalovirus	Pulmonary, gut or CNS infections

Azidothymidine

Although there is no cure for AIDS or ARC, some progress has been made with drugs which suppress the replication of HIV within the host's cells, such as azidothymidine (AZT or Zidovudine).

A double-blind, placebo-controlled trial of AZT in 282 patients with AIDS or ARC showed that the drug can decrease mortality and reduce the frequency of opportunistic infections (Wood and Geddes, 1987). AZT is, however, toxic and many patients in the trial complained of headaches, nausea, myalgia and insomnia. Bone marrow suppression was observed in many, with anaemia necessitating blood transfusions in 24 per cent of cases. AZT is indicated for AIDS patients who have had one episode of *Pneumocystis carinii* pneumonia and for patients with advanced ARC.

Clinical trials are currently in progress with another drug, dideoxycytidine. Cytotoxic therapy and radiotherapy are used for patients with Kaposi's sarcoma, and remission has occurred in a proportion of cases.

Forecasting the spread of AIDS has great potential for error as many individuals infected with the virus have probably not yet come forward for testing. The number of reported cases continues to double at approximately 10-monthly intervals, but the spread into the heterosexual population is not, to date, as great as was forecast.

PNEUMOCYSTIS CARINII

This organism has been associated mainly with outbreaks of disease in neonatal nurseries, the predisposing factors being prematurity and malnourishment. It may also occur in those suffering from an immunological disease, chronic disease or malignancy. Since 1980, *Pneumocystis carinii* pneumonia (PCP) has been a major feature of the acquired immunodeficiency syndrome. It is this infection which often brings the AIDS sufferer to hospital for the first time.

Mode of Spread

The mode of transmission and natural habitat of *Pneumocystis carinii* are unknown and, although small outbreaks have occurred, person-to-person transmission has not been proved.

Symptoms

Presenting symptoms include dyspnoea, anorexia, cough and cyanosis.

Treatment

High dosage of trimethoprim and sulphamethoxazole (combined as Septrin) are recommended. As much as five times the normal dose may be necessary.

CRYPTOSPORIDIUM ENTERIDITIS

This is an intestinal sporozoan parasite first reported to be a cause of gastroenteritis in humans in 1976 and previously only recognised in animals. This is normally a rare, self-limiting diarrhoeal disease but it is one of the opportunistic infections frequently encountered in patients with AIDS (Navin and Juranek, 1984).

Incidence

A total of 9385 reports of cryptosporidium infection have been reported since laboratory reporting began in 1983 (figure 10.3). Outbreaks occur within families, but many are reported from day nurseries, colleges and camp-sites (Communicable Disease Report, 1987c).

The dramatic rise in incidence may be partly due to the development of improved diagnostic methods (Communicable Disease Report, 1988c). Cryptosporidium may

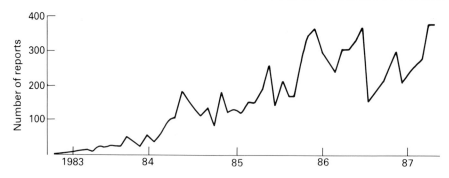

Fig 10.3 Laboratory reports of cryptosporidium infection in England and Wales, 1983–1987 (Reproduced by kind permission of the Communicable Disease Surveillance Centre)

be missed if a routine ova and parasite examination is performed as the oocytes are small and can be overlooked or mistaken for yeasts. Previous tests (before 1978) relied on electron microscopic examination of intestinal biopsies (Ma and Soave, 1982).

Symptoms

Asymptomatic or self-limiting infection occurs in individuals with an intact immune system but, in those with a compromised immune system, particularly AIDS patients, chronic, watery diarrhoea occurs. This is often accompanied by abdominal cramps, nausea and vomiting which may last for 5 to 6 days but, in AIDS patients, can last much longer.

The incubation period is between 3 and 10 days.

Treatment

No drug has been found effective for treatment or prophylaxis, but the disease is self-limiting in otherwise healthy people. However, prevention of transmission in immunocompromised patients is very important.

CRYPTOCOCCUS NEOFORMANS

Cryptococcus neoformans is a soil fungus which can cause pulmonary infection initially through inhalation. It can be found in the sputum of healthy adults. In AIDS or immunocompromised patients it can become disseminated to the meninges or other organs. The increased incidence of cryptococcosis in the UK is directly linked to AIDS (figure 10.4), predominantly causing meningitis, although pneumonia and septicaemia also occur (Communicable Disease Report, 1988d).

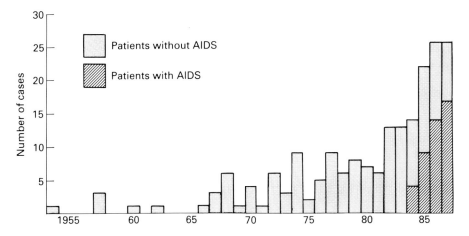

Fig 10.4 Human cryptococcosis in the UK
(Reproduced by kind permission of the Communicable Disease Surveillance Centre)

Incidence

Cryptococcus can be found in the sputum of healthy adults and is commonly found in nature.

Symptoms

In pulmonary infection there is no characteristic clinical picture, although the illness may start with influenza-like symptoms, followed by low grade fever and weight loss.

Invasion of the central nervous system may produce signs of meningitis, meningoencephalitis or a space-occupying lesion. Fifty per cent of patients presenting with cryptococcal meningitis are immunosuppressed or have an underlying disease, e.g. lymphoma or diabetes. Headache is the most frequent symptom, then fever and weight loss, mental aberration and nausea and vomiting. The cerebrospinal fluid pressure may be high and abnormalities on lumbar puncture resemble those of tuberculous meningitis.

Treatment

Although most (non-compromised) patients recover without treatment, and dissemination to the central nervous system is quite rare, treatment is recommended for immunocompromised patients, comprising amphotericin B at a dosage of 0.3 to 1.0 mg/kg/day for six to eight weeks in pulmonary infection (Medoff 1986a).

For cryptococcal meningitis, a drug dose of 0.5 mg/kg of body weight daily is recommended, although it may vary between 0.3 and 1.0 mg/kg depending on the clinical condition. In some instances, it may be necessary to administer the drug intrathecally.

Oral 5-fluorocytosine (5FC) readily penetrates the cerebrospinal fluid; toxic reactions are uncommon. Ketoconazole and miconazole may also be used (Medoff, 1986b).

HEPATITIS B

Four types of hepatitis virus have been described and, although here we are only concerned with hepatitis B, it is important to know the distinction between them (table 10.4). Other viruses, most notably cytomegalovirus and Epstein–Barr virus, have also been shown to cause hepatitis.

Hepatitis B follows a protracted course lasting some weeks to months. The illness is normally self-limiting but a small number of people (fewer than 5 per cent in the UK) may become chronically infected. The liver becomes inflamed with diffuse, patchy hepatocellular necrosis affecting all the liver cells.

Hepatitis B is a stable virus which is not easily destroyed and which can remain viable in the environment for weeks. It is destroyed by:

- Autoclaving at 134°C for a minimum of three minutes
- Boiling for not less than five minutes
- Hypochlorite 1 per cent or gluteraldehyde 2 per cent for 30 minutes

Table 10.4   Classification of hepatitis

	Incubation period	Route of transmission	Incidence	Carrier state
Hepatitis A (HAV)	4–5 weeks	Faeco/oral	Rarely in hospitals	No chronic carrier state
Hepatitis B (HBV)	6 weeks–6 months	Parenteral inoculation of infected blood or by sexual intercourse. Also 'needlestick' injuries	Patients are potential source especially to dentists and surgeons	Can be asymptomatic carriers
Non A, non B hepatitis	Not identified	Parenteral or enteral		Carrier state can occur
Delta hepatitis			Coinfection with hepatitis B	Possible chronic carrier state

Terminology

The World Health Organisation recommends the following terminology for hepatitis:

- *HBV* Hepatitis B virus
- *HBsAg* Hepatitis B surface antigen (Australia antigen)
- *HBcAg* Hepatitis B core antigen
- *HBeAg* The e antigen associated with the core of the whole virus
- *Anti-HBs* Antibody to hepatitis B surface antigen
- *Anti-HBc* Antibody to hepatitis B core antigen
- *Anti-HBe* Antibody to the e antigen
- *HAV* Hepatitis A virus
- *Anti-HAV* Antibody to HAV
- *Non-A, Non-B* This infection may be caused by a number of different agents which have not been identified yet. Serological markers are not available.

Structure

The complete virion is known as a **Dane particle**. Its structure is shown in figure 10.5.

Incidence

The World Health Organisation Expert Health Committee estimates the number of hepatitis B surface antigen carriers throughout the world to be 200 to 280 million. In tropical areas, mainly in Africa, South East Asia and the Far East, the prevalence is high, with carriage rates of up to 20 per cent. Mothers who are carriers transmit the infection to their babies perinatally. These babies become persistent carriers.

The chronic carrier state in the UK is assessed by screening blood donors. It is

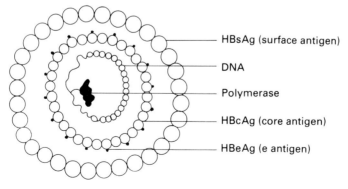

Fig 10.5 Structure of the hepatitis B virion (Dane particle)

approximately 1 in 1000, the rate being twice as high in males, and the predominant age group is in early adult life.

The incidence of acute hepatitis B decreased dramatically over the years 1984 to 1987 (figure 10.6). Polakoff (1983) suggests that, although hepatitis B vaccine has been available for five years, it is unlikely to have been employed widely enough to have produced such a swift change, and that public warnings to intravenous drug abusers who share syringes and needles have caused the drop in acute hepatitis B infection as a side-effect. The advice given to the general public in preventing transmission of HIV by the use of condoms may also have contributed to the reduced incidence of hepatitis B infection through sexual contact.

High incidence of hepatitis B is also found among recipients of many blood transfusions (especially of unscreened blood), haemodialysis or kidney transplant patients and residents of mental handicap institutions, particularly those with Down's syndrome. A defective immune response system gives the latter a tendency to become chronic carriers.

Smith (1987) studied the prevalence rates of hepatitis B in health-care workers using the markers HBsAg, anti-HBs and anti-HBc, which would indicate current and past infections. He demonstrated overall incidences of infection of 1.1 per cent in dental staff, 3.2 per cent in nursing staff and 6 per cent in junior medical staff.

The prevalence of hepatitis B antibodies among London blood donors with no

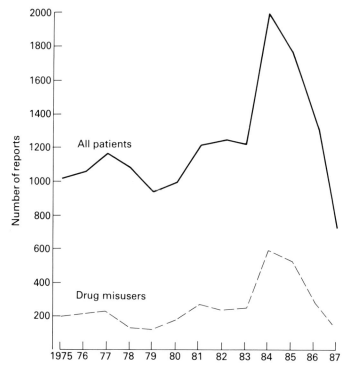

Fig 10.6   Acute hepatitis B reports 1975–1987
(Reproduced by kind permission of the Communicable Disease Surveillance Centre)

history of jaundice has been shown in one study to be 1.6 per cent (Tedder et al, 1980).

Symptoms

Acute hepatitis B infection may go unnoticed or only be associated with non-specific symptoms but, typically, it leads to the appearance of HBsAg (surface antigen) in the blood. The antigen reaches a maximum level when, or just before, the jaundice develops and decreases over the next few weeks as the patient recovers (figure 10.7).

The degree of infection is assessed by looking for e antigen (HBeAg) which may be found in the serum. HBeAg only occurs in the presence of HBsAg and is found transiently, early in acute infections. During the acute phase when e antigen can be detected in the serum, even a very small amount of blood can transmit the disease. Once the antigen is replaced by anti-e antibodies, the risk of transmitting infection is greatly reduced.

Clinical recovery from hepatitis B may take several months, and a bi-phasic illness with resurgence of serum transaminase and bilurubin levels can occur. Approximately 1 per cent of hospitalised patients have rapid clearance of viral antigens (HBsAg and HBeAg) and proceed to fulminant hepatic failure (Fagan, 1987).

Prevention

Prevention of spread of hepatitis B in hospital is dependent on:

● Indentification of infectious cases and safe management of carriers

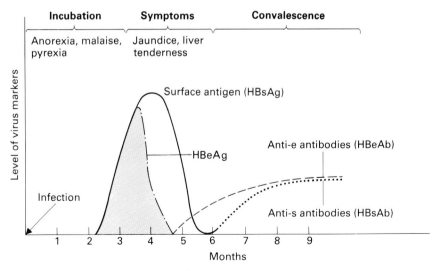

Fig 10.7 Pattern of clinical presentation of hepatitis B

- Appropriate procedures to prevent infection of health-care workers
- Passive immunisation if there is accidental inoculation of infectious material
- Active immunisation of staff likely to be at risk of infection, i.e. laboratory staff, dentists, surgeons, midwives, operating theatre staff, etc.

Blood from a high-risk patient spilled directly onto the hand represents little or no risk but, if it comes into contact with mucous membranes, the eyes or broken skin, the risk will be greater. Faeces, urine and saliva are only infectious if contaminated by blood, and they have not been implicated in hospital transmission.

A clearly written policy is essential for the management of hepatitis B patients, and it must include advice on the safe disposal of 'sharps' and a procedure to follow in the event of needlestick injury (table 10.5). A policy of management in the operating theatre, renal dialysis unit, etc. is needed, including a recommendation that only essential surgery should be performed when the patient is at the highly infectious stage (i.e. if he or she has HbeAg detectable in the blood).

Hepatitis B vaccine is now generally available and can be prescribed by a general practitioner. It is well tolerated with very few side-effects being reported.

Screening of antenatal patients occurs routinely in the UK, but the expense of screening the total population would be unjustified, even for surgical procedures. In NHS hospitals, only those in high-risk groups are screened, although some

Table 10.5 A suggested policy for needlestick injury

1. Wash injured part and encourage bleeding.
2. Report to immediate superior and occupational health department.
3. Nurse in charge/house officer to establish who the needle was used on (the donor) and whether blood has recently been sent to laboratory for other tests, e.g. cross-match, LFTs.
   If no blood specimen is available, the patient's doctor must provide a fresh sample to be sent to virology department as soon as possible.
4. The occupational health department will inform the virology department of the incident, document all results, institute treatment and, if appropriate, follow up.
   A sample from the member of staff (recipient) will be requested by the occupational health department if the donor is HBsAg positive.
5. If the donor is unknown, e.g. needlestick from an over-full 'sharps' bin, the incident must still be reported. The nurse in charge should also inform the occupational health department of any high risk patients in the ward.

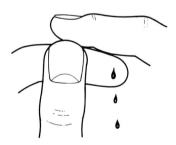

Remember to complete an accident form

All 'sharps' injuries can be prevented by good practice

private hospitals who admit patients from countries where hepatitis B is endemic routinely screen patients on arrival. The high-risk groups are:

- Those with a history of liver disease or suffering from jaundice
- Patients with a history of renal disease, dialysis or kidney transplant
- Those who have had multiple blood transfusions, e.g. haemophiliacs
- Male homosexuals
- Intravenous drug abusers
- Immigrants from high-prevalence countries
- Institutionalised, mentally impaired patients
- People who have heavy tattooing or scarification (tribal marking)
- Babies of infected mothers (these babies are now vaccinated within 48 hours of birth)

Treatment

The clinical course of hepatitis B is variable and there is no specific treatment other than that of rest and alleviation of symptoms. Rest would certainly be advised in severe cases or in the very elderly or frail, but the deleterious effects of exercise, claimed by many, have failed to be confirmed by studies. The outcome of infection is dictated by the individual's response, and his recovery depends on the ability of the immune system to clear the virus.

Except in cases where there is hepatic failure, changing the diet does not appear to affect the outcome. Where there are symptoms of anorexia and nausea and the patient is malnourished, it may be advisable to adopt a high calorie or high protein diet.

Corticosteroids have been found to be favourable for chronic active hepatitis, with liver function tests soon returning to normal, but are not beneficial in severe, acute viral hepatitis.

Interferon has been shown to inhibit the production of Dane particles in persistently infected patients, i.e. those demonstrating HBsAg for more than one year.

Advice is given by the Joint Committee on Vaccination and Immunisation, guided by the Advisory Group on Hepatitis, on which groups of staff and patients should receive priority vaccination (Yellowlees and Poole, 1962).

SUMMARY

There has been a constant ebb and flow of infections and communicable diseases over the last hundred years. New and improved vaccines mean that children are now better protected when first attending school, and BCG (Bacille–Calmette–Guerin) vaccination for tuberculosis may become unnecessary, at least in the UK, as has smallpox vaccination.

Protection afforded to health-care workers against hepatitis B should reduce the occupational hazard, particularly to high-risk groups such as dentists and surgeons. It also has implications for the male homosexual population and the increasing number of intravenous drug abusers.

Efforts to control the dramatic and serious epidemic of AIDS continues to be focused on its prevention. Although some measure of success has been recorded in slowing down the disease with azidothymidine (AZT), we may have to wait some years for a vaccine. Predicting the incidence of AIDS is complicated by the possibility that the available HIV seropositivity data might be an underestimate of the true incidence. However, the care needed for these patients will be concentrated in the community, with hospitalisation at intervals for treatment of opportunistic infections. Increasing demands for hospice care and continuing-care teams will be experienced.

Food-borne salmonellosis and campylobacter infections continue to increase in developed countries, mainly communicated in poultry and meat, and the UK government may consider the possible irradiation of poultry before retailing. There has been a recent increase in salmonellosis from products containing raw egg (e.g. ice cream and mayonnaise) and in those who eat raw eggs, such as body builders. It has also been reported where raw eggs have been included in nasogastric feeds (Communicable Disease Report, 1988e).

The changing patterns of communicable disease are often the result of changing trends in human behaviour. Legionnaires' disease is not a new disease, but man's efforts to adjust his environment allowed a previously non-pathogenic organism to reach susceptible hosts. It was with this in mind that, in the planning of the new Inverclyde Royal Hospital, water-cooled towers were discarded and replaced by an air-cooled system, despite the higher running costs of the latter. It could be that architects and planners will in the future follow suit.

Although the incidence of insect- and parasite-borne disease has been dramatically reduced in developed countries with the help of insecticides and public health measures, a new infection has been reported in the UK, predominately in the south east of England, as a result of increased enthusiasm for watersports. A severe itchy rash was found to be caused by cercaria, a parasite of the giant pond snail. It would seem that this type of problem will need to be included in health education of the future.

This chapter has looked at some of the major changes in microbiological behaviour. It is the responsibility of each health-care worker to keep abreast of the constant changing pattern of infections and communicable diseases. Change is inevitable and perpetual; microbiology is a dynamic science.

References

Abbott J D, Hepner E D and Clifford C (1980) Salmonella infections in hospital. A report from the Public Health Laboratory Service Salmonella Subcommittee. *Journal of Hospital Infection*, **1**: 307–314.

Adler M W (1986) Time for honest talk about AIDS. *The Times*, July 8.

Allen J and Mellin G (1982) The new epidemic immune deficiency, opportunistic infections and Kaposi's sarcoma. *American Journal of Nursing*, **82**(11): 1718–1722.

Baldry P E (1976) *The Battle against Bacteria, A Fresh Look*. London: Cambridge University Press.

Bolton R P (1980) Vancomycin dose for pseudomembranous colitis (letter). *Lancet*, **ii**: 428.

Bradley J M, Noone P, Townsend D E and Gribb W B (1985) Methicillin resistant *Staphylococcus aureus* in a London hospital. *Lancet*, **i**: 1493–1495.

British Dental Association (1987) *Guide to Blood Borne Viruses and the Control of Cross Infection in Dentistry*. London: British Dental Association.

Butzler J P, Dekeyser P, Detrain M and Dethen F (1973) Related vibrio in stools. *Journal of Paediatrics*, **82**: 493.

Cartwright K A V (1987) Meningoccal disease in Gloucestershire: The Stonehouse Survey. *PHLS Microbiology Digest*, **4**(4): 1–2.

Cartwright K A V, Stuart J M and Noah N D (1986) An outbreak of meningococcal disease in Gloucestershire. *Lancet*, **ii**: 561.

Communicable Disease Report (1981) Meningococcal infection – chemoprophylaxis. *Communicable Disease Report*, **81**/12: 1.

Communicable Disease Report (1986) Foodborne disease surveillance in England and Wales 1984. *Communicable Disease Report*, **86**/34: 3–6.

Communicable Disease Report (1987a) Group A meningococcal meningitis: Middle East. *Communicable Disease Report*, **87**/35: 1.

Communicable Disease Report (1987b) Legionnaires' Disease, Yugoslavia. *Communicable Disease Report*, **87**/40: 1.

Communicable Disease Report (1987c) Cryptosporidium surveillance. *Communicable Disease Report*, **87**/45: 1.

Communicable Disease Report (1987d) Acute meningococcal infections. *Communicable Disease Report*, **87**/50: 1.

Communicable Disease Report (1988a) Legionella outbreak: Portland Place, London. *Communicable Disease Report*, **88**/18: 1.

Communicable Disease Report (1988b) AIDS: United Kingdom: 1982 – April 1988. *Communicable Disease Report*, **88**/18: 3.

Communicable Disease Report (1988c) Cryptosporidium surveillance. *Communicable Disease Report*, **88**/20: 2.

Communicable Disease Report (1988d) Cryptococcosis: before and during the AIDS era. *Communicable Disease Report*, **88**/20: 3.

Communicable Disease Report (1988e) Salmonella enteritidis surveillance. *Communicable Disease Report*, **88**/34: 1.

Cooke E M and Marples R R (1985) Outbreak of staphylococcal infection. *PHLS Microbiology Digest*, **2**: 62–64.

Cookson B D, Webster M, Talsania H and Phillips I (1987) The eradication and subsequent control of an epidemic methicillin-resistant *Staphylococcus aureus* (EMRSA) in two hospitals. Poster presentation, 1st International Conference of the Hospital Infection Society, London.

Crossley K, Landesman B and Zaske D (1979). An outbreak of infection caused by a strain of staph aureus resistant to methicillin and aminoglycoside, II. Epidemiologic studies. *Journal of Infectious Disease*, **1139**: 280–287.

Department of Health and Social Security (1986) *The Report of the Committee of Inquiry into an Outbreak of Food Poisoning at Stanley Royd Hospital*. London: HMSO.

Department of Health and Social Security (1987a) *Engineering Note 4: Cooling Towers and Evaporative Condensers*. HN (87) 16. London: DHSS.

Department of Health and Social Security (1987b) *Engineering Guidance Note 5: Hot and Cold Water Distribution Systems*. HN (87) 17. London: DHSS.

Doenges J L (1939) Spirochaetes in the gastric glands of Macacus rhesus and of man without related disease. *Archives of Pathology*, **27**: 469–477.

Donta S T and Myers M G (1982) *Clostridium difficile* toxin in asymptomatic neonates. *Journal of Paediatrics*, **100**: 431–434.

Edelstein P H (1986). Control of Legionella in hospitals. *Journal of Hospital Infection*, **8**: 109–115.

Fagan E (1987) Hepatitis caused by hepatitis B virus. *The Practitioner*, **231**: 371–378.

Fisher Hoch S P, Bartlett C L R, Tobin J O'H, Gillett M B, Nelson A M, Pritchard J E, Smith M G, Swann R A, Talbot J M and Thom J A (1981) Investigations and control of an outbreak of Legionnaires' disease in a district general hospital. *Lancet*, **i**: 932–936.

Gardner A M N, Stamp M, Bowgen J A and Moore B (1962) The Infection Control Sister, a new member of the Infection Control Team in general hospital. *Lancet*, **ii**: 710–711.

Geberding J L and Henderson D K (1987) Design of rational infection control policies for human immunodeficiency virus infection. *Journal of Infectious Disease*, **156**(6): 861–864.

Hafiz S, McEntegart M G, Martin R S and Waitkin S A (1975) Clostridium difficile in the urogenital tract of males and females. *Lancet*, **i**: 420–421.

Health and Safety Commission (1985) *Guidance on Handling Hepatitis B Specimens in Clinical Laboratories*. London: HMSO.

Helms C M, Massanari R M, Zeitler R, Streed S, Gilchrist J R, Hall N, Hausler W J, Sywasink J, Johnson W, Wintermeyer L and Hierholzer W J Jr (1983) Legionnaires' disease associated with a hospital water system: a cluster of 24 nosocomial cases. *Annals of Internal Medicine*, **99**: 172.

Kappas A, Shinagawa N, Arabi Y, Thompson H, Burdon D W, Dimock F, George R H, Alexander Williams J and Keighley M R B (1978) Diagnosis of pseudomembranous colitis. *British Medical Journal*, **1**: 675–678.

Keighley M R B, Burdon D W, Arabi Y, Alexander Williams J, Thompson H, Youngs D, Johnson M, Bentley S, George R H and Mogg G A G (1978) Randomised controlled trial of vancomycin for pseudomembranous colitis and post-operative diarrhoea. *British Medical Journal*, **2**: 1667–1669.

Kim K H, Fekety R, Batts D H, Brown D, Cudmore M, Siwach J and Waters D (1981) Isolation of Clostridium difficile from the environment and contacts of patients with antibiotic associated colitis. *Journal of Infectious Disease*, **143**(1): 42–49.

Larson H E, Parry J V, Price A B, Davies D R, Dolby J and Tyrrell D A J (1977) Undescribed toxin in pseudomembranous colitis. *British Medical Journal*, **1**: 1246–1248.

Locksley R M, Cohen M L, Quinn T C, Tomkins L S, Coyle M B, Kirahara J M and Counts G W (1982) Multiply antibiotic-resistant *Staphylococcus aureus* introduction, transmission and evolution of nosocomial infection. *Annals of Internal Medicine*, **97**(3): 317–324.

Lombardo J (1988) HIV–1 testing: an overview. *International Clinical Products Review*; Jan/Feb 88: 14–24.

Ma P and Soave R (1982) Three step stool examination for cryptosporidiosis in 10 homosexual men with protracted watery diarrhoea. *Journal of Infectious Disease*, **147**: 824–828.

Medoff G (1986a) Cryptococcal meningitis. In: *Infectious Diseases and Medical Microbiology*, ed. Braude A I, pp. 1072–1073. Philadelphia: W B Saunders.

Medoff G (1986b) Pulmonary cryptococcosis. In: *Infectious Diseases and Medical Microbiology*, ed. Braude A I, pp. 853–858. Philadelphia: W B Saunders.

Miller D, Weber J and Green J (1986) *The management of AIDS patients*. London: Macmillan.

Navin T R and Jarunek D O (1984) Cryptosporidiosis; clinical, epidemiological and parasitological review. *Review of Infectious Diseases*, **6**: 31.

Nightingale F (1863) *Notes on Hospitals*. London: Longman.

PHLS Salmonella Sub Committee (1983) *Notes on Control of Human Sources of Gastrointestinal Infection, Infestations and Bacterial Intoxications*. London: PHLS.

Pinching A J (1986) AIDS and Africa; lessons for us all. *Journal of the Royal Society of Medicine*, **79**(9): 501–3.

Polakoff S (1988) Decrease in acute hepatitis B incidence continued in 1987. *Communicable Disease Report*, **88/05**: 1.

Price E H (1984) *Staphylococcus epidermidis* infection in cerebrospinal fluid shunts. *Journal of Hospital Infection*, **5**: 7–17.

Royal College of Nursing Working Party (1987) *Introduction to Hepatitis B and Nursing Guidelines for Infection Control*. London: Royal College of Nursing.

Royal College of Nursing Working Party (1987) *AIDS Nursing Guidelines*. London: Royal College of Nursing.

Rutala W A, Katz E B S, Sheretz R J and Sarubbi F A Jr (1983) Environmental study of methicillin resistant staph aureus epidemic in a burns unit. *Journal of Clinical Microbiology*, **18**: 683–688.

Sebald M and Veron M (1963) Teneur en bases de l'ADN et classification des vibrions. *Annales de l'Institute Pasteur*, **105**: 897–910.

Selkon J B, Stokes E R and Ingham H R (1980). *Journal of Hospital Infection*, **1**(1): 41–46.

Shanson D C (1982) *Microbiology in Clinical Practice*. Bristol: John Wright.

Sim A J W and Dudley H A F (1988) Surgeons and HIV. *British Medical Journal*, **1**: 80.

Skirrow M B (1977) Campylobacter enteritis; a 'new' disease. *British Medical Journal*, **2**: 9–11.

Smith C E T (1987) A study of the prevalence of markers of hepatitis B infection in hospital staff. *Journal of Hospital Infection*, **9**: 39–42.

Sullivan M, Sheretz R, Reuma P and Russell B (1984) Simultaneous *Staphylococcus aureus* nursery outbreaks in a community and a University hospital traced to one nurse. Paper presented at the 11th Annual Meeting of the Association for Practitioners in Infection Control, Washington DC.

Svedhem A (1980) Campylobacter jejuni-enteritis transmitted from cat to man. *Lancet*, **i**: 713–4.

Tiehan W and Vogt R L (1978) Waterborne Campylobacter enteritis. Vermont. *Morbidity and Mortality*, **27**: 207.

Treloar A J and Kalra L, (1987) Mortality and *Clostridium difficile* diarrhoea in the elderly. *Lancet*, **ii**: 1279.

Waghorn D J (1987) Campylobacter pylorides; a new organism to explain an old problem? *Postgraduate Medical Journal*, **63**: 533–537.

Ward T T, Winn R E, Hartstein A I and Sewell D L (1981) Observations relating to an inter-hospital outbreak of MRSA: role of antimicrobial therapy in infection control. *Infection Control*, **2**: 453–459.

Wells N (1986) *The AIDS Virus; Forecasting its Impact*. London: Office of Health Economics.

White A (1961) Relation between quantitative nasal culture and dissemination of staphylococci. *Journal of Laboratory Clinical Medicine*, **58**: 273–277.

Wood M J and Geddes A M (1987) Antiviral therapy. *Lancet*, **ii**: 1189–1191.

Yellowlees H and Poole A A B (1962) *Hepatitis B Vaccine, Guidance on Use*, CNO (82) 11 and CNO (82) 13. London: HMSO.

Zar F, Geisler J and Brown V A (1985) Asymptomatic carriage of cryptosporidium in the stool of a patient with acquired immunodeficiency syndrome. *Journal of Infectious Disease*, **151**: 195.

Further Reading

Baldry P E (1976) *The Battle against Bacteria: A Fresh Look*. London: Cambridge University Press.

Bradley J M, Noone P, Townsend D E and Grubb W B, (1985) Methicillin resistant *Staphylococcus aureus* in a London hospital. *Lancet*, **i**: 1493–1495.

Daniels V (1985) *AIDS and the Acquired Immune Deficiency Syndrome*. Lancaster: MTP Press.

Editorial (1986) Clostridium difficile: a neglected pathogen in chronic care wards. *Lancet*, **ii**: 790–791.

Guidelines for the control of epidemic methicillin resistant *Staphylococcus aureus*. Report of a combined working part of the Hospital Infection Society and the British Society for Antimicrobial Therapy (1986) *Journal of Hospital Infection*, **7**(2): 193–202.

Miller D, Weber J and Green J (1986) *The Management of AIDS Patients*. London: Macmillan.

Shanson D C (1982) *Microbiology in Clinical Practice*. Bristol: John Wright.

Appendix I
Routes of Transmission of
Important Infections

Infection	Causative organism	Reservoir	Entry route	Exit route	Mode of spread to other patients
Acquired immune deficiency syndrome (AIDS)	Human immunodeficiency virus (HIV)	Infected person or carrier	Blood stream Neonate: via placenta or across mucosal membrane during birth Adult: inoculation damage skin/mucous membranes (particularly genitourinary)	Blood, semen; low level of virus in other body fluids	Equipment or articles contaminated with blood. Staff themselves may be at risk from needlestick injuries or splashes of blood into the eye
Anthrax ● Cutaneous	Bacillus anthracis	Infected animal hides and furs Contaminated soil	Skin (direct contact)	Skin lesions	Staff hands/equipment/ articles contaminated by vesicle discharge
● Pulmonary (wool sorters' disease)			Respiratory tract (inhalation of spores)	Respiratory tract secretions	Airborne/droplet spread of secretions of respiratory tract. Strict isolation
Brucellosis	Brucella abortus	Tissues, blood, urine and aborted foetuses of infected animals. Raw milk from infected animals	Skin (direct contact) Ingestion	Usually none Occasionally via urine	No evidence of person-to-person spread for either brucella infection
(Undulant and Malta fevers)	Brucella meltensis	Raw milk from infected animals	Ingestion		
Candidiasis (thrush) of mouth, skin, septic fingers, vagina; systemic candidiasis	Candida albicans	Man. Normal flora of mouth, vagina and intestines	Damaged tissue Endogenous in compromised host	Exudates	Spread particularly to compromised patients by staff hands or equipment contaminated by infectious exudates

Infection	Causative organism	Reservoir	Entry route	Exit route	Mode of spread to other patients
Chickenpox	Varicella zoster virus	Infected person	Respiratory tract (inhalation)	Respiratory tract secretions Skin lesions	Airborne/droplet spread of secretions of respiratory tract and lesions Staff hands/equipment/articles contaminated by vesicle discharge
Cholera	Vibrio cholerae	Water contaminated by faeces or vomit from cases. May be natural environmental reservoir	Alimentary tract (ingestion)	Faeces and vomit	Staff hands/equipment/articles contaminated with infectious faeces or vomit
Cytomegalovirus ● Neonatal	Cytomegalovirus	Infected person	Blood stream in utero. Contact with cervical excretions during delivery	Urine, saliva, cervical excretions, breast milk, semen	Staff hands/equipment/articles contaminated with infectious urine or saliva
● Children: hepatitis ● Adult: inapparent glandular fever type or general infection in compromised host			Blood stream. May be endogenous in compromised host – this is a reactivation of previous infection	Urine and saliva	
Diphtheria	Corynebacterium diphtheriae	Infected person	Respiratory tract Local lesion	Respiratory secretions Exudate from lesions	Airborne/droplet spread of secretions of respiratory tract Staff hands/equipment/articles contaminated by secretions

Infection	Causative organism	Reservoir	Entry route	Exit route	Mode of spread to other patients
Dysentery					
● Amoebic	*Entamoeba histolytica*	Man – usually a chronically ill or asymptomatic cyst carrier	Alimentary tract Ingestion of contaminated water or food	Faeces	Infection not initiated in temperature climate. Elsewhere – staff hands/ equipment/articles contaminated by faeces
● Bacilliary	Shigella spp.	Infected person	Alimentary tract (ingestion)	Faeces	Very easily spread by staff hands/equipment/articles contaminated by faeces
Gastrointestinal infections	*Salmonella* spp. *Clostridium perfringens* (toxin) *Campylobacter jejuni* *Staphylococcus aureus* (toxin) *Enteropathogenic E. coli* (infants)	Infected person or carrier	Alimentary tract (ingestion)	Faeces	Contaminated staff hands/ and equipment. In neonates spread may occur easily via contaminated equipment, e.g. rectal thermometers
	Rotavirus (infants)		Respiratory tract, alimentary tract		Rotavirus may spread via faecal respiratory routes
Glandular fever (infectious mononucleosis)	Epstein–Barr virus	Infected person	Mucous membranes of mouth	Saliva	Very close contact required for transmission. Infants may be infected by contaminated staff hands
Gonococcal infection	*Neisseria gonorrhoea*	Infected person			
● Genitourinary tract			Genitourinary mucous membranes	Discharge from urethra and vagina	Sexual contact only
● Secondary arthritis			May be secondary spread via blood stream	None	
● Ophthalmia neonatorum			Contact of eyes with infected cervical excretions during childbirth	Conjunctival discharges	Spread to neonates by staff hands/equipment contaminated with conjunctival discharge

Infection	Causative organism	Reservoir	Entry route	Exit route	Mode of spread to other patients
Haemolytic streptococcal infection	Haemolytic streptococcus. There are 14 Lancefield groups of streptococcus (A–O). Groups A, C and G are usually responsible for human streptococcal infections	Human cases and throat and nasal carriers. Vaginal carriage in neonatal infections	Upper respiratory tract		Airborne. Staff hands/equipment/articles contaminated by infectious secretions
● Tonsillitis				Respiratory secretions	
● Otitis media				Aural and respiratory secretions	
● Meningitis				None	
● Secondary pneumonia				Sputum	
● Scarlet fever				Exudate from lesions and respiratory secretions	
● Erysipelas cellulitis, wound infection			Damaged skin	Exudate from lesions	
● Puerperal sepsis			Locally at placental site	Lochia	
Secondary infections Rheumatic fever and acute nephritis may occur but are not transmissible					

Infection	Causative organism	Reservoir	Entry route	Exit route	Mode of spread to other patients
Hepatitis (viral)					
● Hepatitis A	Hepatitis A virus	Infected person	Alimentary tract Ingestion of contaminated water or food	Faeces, urine	Staff hands/equipment/ articles contaminated with infectious faeces or urine
● Hepatitis B	Hepatitis B virus	Infected person or carrier	Blood stream Neonate: via placenta or across mucosal membrane during birth Adult: inoculation damaged skin or mucous membranes	Blood Saliva, semen and other body fluids in acute stage	Staff hands/equipment/ articles contaminated with blood. Other body fluids in acute stage Staff themselves may be at risk from needle-stick injuries or splashes of blood into the eye
Herpes simplex	Herpes simplex virus				
● Type I (oral herpes) Primary infection: symptomless, gingivostomatitis or conjunctivitis. May remain as latent infection Herpetic whitlow		Infected person	Direct contact with mucosa Damaged skin	Exudate from infected lesions	Contaminated staff hands/ equipment/articles particularly in the care of infants or patients with eczema (Staff should wear gloves for their own protection and to avoid spread)
● Type II (genital herpes)			Genitourinary mucous membranes during coitus	Exudate from genital lesions	

Infection	Causative organism	Reservoir	Entry route	Exit route	Mode of spread to other patients
Herpes zoster (shingles)	Herpes zoster virus	Man	Virus latent in nerve cells following chickenpox infection	Skin lesions	Will spread to cause chickenpox by airborne spread or staff hands/equipment/articles contaminated with vesicle fluid. Important to protect compromised patients
Malaria	Plasmodium vivax P. malariae P. falciparum	Man. The female anopheline mosquito can act as intermediate reservoir	Blood stream usually following mosquito bite or blood transfusion	Blood	Not directly transmitted
Meningitis (meningococcal meningitis)	Neisseria meningitidis	Infected persons or carriers	Respiratory tract. Close contact with nasopharyngeal carriers required	Nasal secretions	Airborne droplet spread. Close contact required
Mumps	Paromyxovirus (measles and respiratory syncytial virus are members of the same virus and are spread by similar routes)	Infected person	Respiratory tract	Respiratory secretions	Airborne droplet spread. Staff hands/equipment/articles contaminated with infected secretions of nose and throat
Poliomyelitis (infantile paralysis)	Polio virus types 1, 2, and 3 (type 1 is the most paralytogenic)	Infected people, often carriers	Alimentary tract (ingestion)	Faeces, pharyngeal secretions	Staff hands/equipment contaminated with infectious faeces or secretions

Infection	Causative organism	Reservoir	Entry route	Exit route	Mode of spread to other patients
Rubella (German measles)	Rubella virus	Infected person	Respiratory tract	Respiratory secretions. Urine and faeces in congenital cases	Airborne droplet spread. Staff hands/articles contaminated by discharge from nose and throat, or urine and faeces in the newborn
Staphylococcal infection	Staphylococcus aureus	Infected person or carrier			Airborne
● Boils, carbuncles, whitlows, impetigo, wound infections		Infections may be endogenous	Damaged skin	Pus from lesions	Staff hands/equipment/articles contaminated by the organism
● Deep abscesses			Damaged skin	Pus after incision	
● Osteomyelitis			Blood stream	Pus after incision	
● Otitis media			Respiratory tract	Discharge from ear	
● Pneumonia			Respiratory tract	Sputum	
● Toxic vomiting (food poisoning)			Alimentary tract (ingestion of contaminated food)	Faeces and vomit	
● Septicaemia			From skin or deep infection	None (excluding initial lesion)	
Syphilis	Trepona pallidum	Infected person			Generally spread by sexual contact
● Congenital			Placenta	Secretions of respiratory tract (nasal and lung lesion)	
● Primary syphilis (chancre)			Skin or mucous membranes during coitis	Discharge from chancre	(Staff should wear gloves to avoid direct contact with lesions in untreated cases)
● Secondary syphilis			Via blood stream	Discharge from surface lesions, e.g. mouth ulcer	
● Tertiary syphilis				Discharge from surface gumma	

Infection	Causative organism	Reservoir	Entry route	Exit route	Mode of spread to other patients
Tuberculosis ● Pulmonary ● Cervical	*Mycobacterium tuberculosis*	Infected person Diseased cattle in bovine tuberculosis (rare)	Respiratory tract	Sputum, discharging sinus	Airborne/droplet spread of bacilli in sputum only
● Alimentary tract			Alimentary tract by ingestion of contaminated milk	Faeces	Occasionally spread by contaminated staff hands/equipment/articles or dust
● Miliary tuberculosis ● Meningitis ● Bone and joint lesions			May be secondary spread via lymphatics and blood stream	Any open lesion	
● Kidney lesions				Urine	
● Testicular lesions					
● Fallopian tube and uterine lesions				Menstrual fluid	
Urinary tract infection (particularly in catheterised patients)	Main cause, Gram-negative bacilli, e.g. *E. coli*, proteus	Patients' faecal flora Staff hands or equipment may act as temporary reservoir	Via urethra	Urine	Staff hands/equipment contaminated by infected urine
Whooping cough (pertussis)	*Bordetella pertussis*	Infected person	Respiratory tract	Respiratory secretions	Airborne droplet spread of infected discharges from respiratory mucous membranes. Staff hands/equipment/articles contaminated by discharges from nose and throat

Infection	Causative organism	Reservoir	Entry route	Exit route	Mode of spread to other patients
Wound infection	*Staphylococcus aureus* *Streptococcus pyogenes*	Both found among patient's own skin and nasal flora or in staff or patient carriers Dust	Damaged skin	Wound exudate and contaminated skin scales	Contaminated hands or clothing of staff. Carriage by staff or other patients, particularly if resistant strain. Airborne dispersal from infected wound or carriage site
	Gram-negative bacilli, e.g. *E. coli* or anaerobes, e.g. bacteroides spp.	Patient's own faecal flora	Damaged skin	Wound exudate	Spread via contamination of staff hands/equipment may occur but is not usually a problem

Appendix II

Parasitic Infestation

of the Skin

The incidence of skin infestation in the UK appears to have diminished over the past two decades. The condition is often accompanied by great distress and embarrassment, which are increased by the fact that infestation is uncommonly seen, especially in acute hospitals. There is evidence that conditions such as scabies and pediculosis capitis are on the increase again in many parts of the world (Maunder, 1983). Knowledge of the nature of the infestation and its mode of spread will enable nurses to treat affected patients confidently.

SCABIES

Infestation by the mite *Sarcoptes scabeii* produces a sensitisation or allergic reaction in the host, giving rise to an intensely itchy rash.

Sarcoptes Scabeii

The male mite is only half the size of the female and is rarely seen (Kirby, 1986). The female mite is 0.3–0.5 mm long and burrows horizontally under the outermost, horny layer of skin, advancing approximately 0.5–5.0 mm per day. The life-span of the mite is six to eight weeks, and her time is spent in the burrow where she lays two or three eggs per day. The eggs hatch in three or four days and the larvae make their way to the surface of the skin. After three moults, and over 10 to 12 days, they mature as adults. Impregnation of the females then starts the cycle again.

The mite moves slowly and requires fairly prolonged contact to transfer to a new host. This may explain why scabies is often seen among children and in patients in long-stay geriatric and psychiatric hospitals, where hand-holding is common. It is unlikely that normal social contact results in the spread of scabies, but close or intimate family contact, especially between bed-fellows or sexual partners, commonly leads to spread.

The burrows are between 15 and 30 cm long and appear as whitish, irregular lines which are diagnostic of scabies. They contain eggs and faeces from the mite, the adult female being just visible as a brownish–white speck at the inner end. Most burrows are found around the anterior aspects of the wrists and between the fingers, although they can sometimes be found around the nipples in women, the penis in men, feet, axillae, groins, elbows and the lower part of the buttocks.

Sensitisation to the mite takes several weeks, during which time the person, although unaware of the presence of the mite, is an infection risk to others. Sensitisation results in an intense itch, skin eruptions and lesions caused by the body's allergic response to the presence of the scabies mite living on and in the upper epidermis.

The site of the itch does not always correspond to the position of the mites, and tends to occur on the hands, arms, legs, inner thighs, sides of the body and around the waist (Maunder, 1983). The itching is worse at night, possibly due to the increased warmth of the bedclothes. The rash may be mistaken for other skin conditions, for example eczema. In the presence of a generalised, irritating rash, therefore, scabies should always be considered and excluded prior to making an alternative diagnosis.

After an initial sensitisation, the reaction to subsequent infections is much quicker, often within a few hours. This results in removal of the mite by scratching before it has had a chance to burrow or become established. This scratching can lead to secondary infection.

Norwegian (Crusted) Scabies

While the average number of adult female mites present in the usual infestation is 12, in **Norwegian** or **crusted** scabies mites are found in large numbers all over the body. As the degree of infectivity is related directly to the number of mites, the infectivity of crusted scabies is much greater than that of the usual infection.

Norwegian scabies is caused by the same mite as simple scabies but, due to a deficiency of the immune system, whether natural or following immunosuppressive drugs, there is no control exercised by the body to limit the number of mites. These multiply rapidly and cover the whole surface of the body. The skin is dry, and crusts appear which are heavily contaminated with mites.

Sufferers, their clothes and bedding constitute a risk to others and it is necessary to wear gloves when handling patients and bedding, to disinfect all clothes and linen and to check contacts for scabies. Fortunately, unless the contacts also have an immune deficiency, they will only develop simple scabies if infested (Robinson, 1986). Precautions prescribed for crusted scabies are unnecessary for a simple case of scabies.

Diagnosis

A clinical diagnosis of scabies can be made when burrows are identified; once seen, they will subsequently be easily recognised. An absolute diagnosis is made after finding the mite. If a needle is used gently to lift the horny layer of the skin, the mite can be removed on the needle-point. To identify a burrow, a marker pen can be rubbed over the suspected area and the ink immediately wiped off with a pad soaked in alcohol. The burrow should absorb some of the ink and show up as a wavering line.

Finding the mite has the additional advantage of encouraging the patient who has seen it to adhere conscientiously to the treatment regimen.

Treatment

Recommended Preparations Available

The recommended products for treatment are:

- 1 per cent gamma benzene hexachloride (e.g. Lindane)
- 0.5 per cent malathion (e.g. Derbac-M liquid)

These are now used in preference to benzyl benzoate which is very irritant to the skin. Gamma benzene hexachloride is contraindicated for infants, nursing and pregnant mothers and those who are severely underweight (Robinson, 1986).

Regimen

Bathing is not necessary before application of the scabicide but, if it is performed for hygienic purposes, the skin must be thoroughly dried and allowed to cool before treatment. Flushed skin (with dilated blood vessels) increases the potential risk of toxicity from the scabicide preparation and decreases its efficacy by conveying it away from the site of infestation.

The prescribed preparation must be applied to all areas of the skin from the neck down, including the soles of the feet. In nursing infants, the face and head should also be treated. Staff should wear gloves to prevent close skin-to-skin contact during the treatment period. The scabicide should be applied with swabs, paying particular attention to the skin folds and discarding the swabs after each application. A single application is usually sufficient to effect a cure. Following treatment, the patient should dress in clean clothes.

If the skin is washed within a certain time after treatment has been carried out, e.g. 24 hours, the lotion should be reapplied. This is particularly important if the hands have been washed.

All family members and other close contacts should be treated at the same time whether or not they are obviously infected. Failure to adhere to this rule can result in the problem being prolonged.

If a patient is cared for over a long period prior to a diagnosis of scabies being made, or if the patient has crusted scabies, involved nursing staff and their spouses should also be offered treatment. In addition, it may be appropriate for all patients in the vicinity of a case of crusted scabies to be given care.

Itching may continue for some time after a successful treatment regimen has been completed. This is due to the allergic reaction and can be treated with calamine lotion.

PEDICULOSIS

Pediculosis results from infestation by the human louse, *Pediculus humanus*. Three conditions are described:

1. **Pediculosis corporis** caused by the body louse, *Pediculus humanus humanus*
2. **Pediculosis capitis** caused by the head louse, *Pediculus humanus capitis*
3. **Pediculosis pubis** caused by the pubic or 'crab' louse, otherwise known as *Phthirus pubis*.

Pediculosis Corporis

Pediculosis corporis is an allergic reaction to the saliva of the body louse as it bites, or to its powdery faeces. The body louse lives in clothing seams in which it lays its adherent eggs. There may be as many as 200 or 300 of these during its three to four week life-span.

The louse visits the body two or three times a day for blood, which it obtains by biting the areas in closest contact with the underclothes, i.e. the shoulders and upper part of the buttocks. The bite results in a small, red macule which is very itchy. Irritation causes scratching, and typical linear scratch marks on the shoulders are almost diagnostic of pediculosis corporis.

Sensitisation follows the initial irritation, with the additional symptoms of a generalised rash, sneezing and eye-watering – the proverbial case of 'feeling lousy' (Maunder, 1980).

Pediculosis corporis is an infestation related to poverty when accompanied by a hostel life of overcrowding and vagrancy. Spread can be directly from the infested person's clothing to the new host or his clothing. As normal laundering of garments will kill the louse, establishment on a new host depends on that person's standard of hygiene. The louse can only transfer in darkness, so handling infected clothing in bright light further reduces the risk of transmission.

Treatment

Treatment of pediculosis corporis need not go further than:

● Hygiene of body and clothing
● Symptomatic treatment to relieve irritation

Typhus, **trench** and **relapsing** fevers are diseases spread by the body louse in some countries, with an increased incidence during outbreaks of war. Typhus fever results from infection of a cut with the louse's faeces, and relapsing fever from infection from the blood of the louse.

Pediculosis Capitis

Pediculosis capitis or head louse infection is, as its name suggests, confined to the head. The areas most commonly colonised are the crown of the head, the hair-line (in particular behind the ears) and the nape of the neck.

The incidence of pediculosis capitis infection is still surprisingly high. In some UK industrial and deprived areas, it may occur in as much as 20 per cent of the population. There also appears to be an increase in the number of cases of head louse infection among middle class children, being more common in any case in children than adults.

It used to be thought that long hair attracted the head louse. This is not borne out in practice, as many children and adults with short hair acquire pediculosis capitis. It would seem reasonable, however, to assume that the route to the scalp is much easier for the louse on short hair than long.

Spread is by direct contact, no matter how brief. This puts the nurse caring for the patient at considerable risk, especially if the condition has not been recognised. Pediculosis capitis is the only pediculosis infection which a carer is liable to catch.

Shiny, pearl-coloured, oval eggs are contained in a cup-shaped receptacle, glued to the base of a hair close to the scalp with a clear, quick-setting secretion from the female louse's accessory glands (Saunders, 1984). The eggs hatch between six and 16 days later and mature during the next eight to 18 days.

Once the egg has hatched, its shell remains firmly glued to the hair shaft, becomes brilliant white in colour and is known as a **nit**. The nit can be removed only from the end of the hair.

Irritation follows hypersensitivity to the saliva and/or faeces of the louse. This leads to scratching and secondary infection which can be extensive, covering not only the scalp but also the face and eyes. Enlarged cervical and posterior auricular glands may occur.

Treatment

The preparations available to treat pediculosis capitis are:

- 0.5 per cent malathion lotion (Prioderm)
- 0.5 per cent carbaryl lotion

The scalp should be soaked with Prioderm solution which is left on overnight, or for at least 12 hours, to dry. A hair dryer must not be used to dry the lotion on the head.

As chlorine will destroy the effect of the lotion, swimming is not allowed for 24 hours after treatment. The hair should be washed thoroughly and dried before treatment if the sufferer has been swimming within the previous 72 hours.

After the lotion has been left overnight, the hair is shampooed and combed. Fine-tooth combing is occasionally recommended by some care-workers although it can be painful, especially on long or neglected hair. The fine-tooth comb would appear to be used far less frequently, in favour of daily care with an ordinary comb.

As head lice are unable to regenerate their injured tissue, the damage caused to them by contact with an ordinary comb is always fatal.

All likely contacts should be treated. According to Maunder (1980), head lice found on pillows and linens 'constitute no danger and no special laundry precautions are needed'. The habit of examining for head lice all those admitted to hospital is sometimes still recommended, particularly in paediatric wards. Treatment of secondary infection may be necessary with either systemic or topical antibiotics.

Shampoos containing malathion or carbaryl are also available, but are not considered as effective as the agents themselves due to the dilution effect and the fact that repeated applications are required. However, they may be of some value during an outbreak of infection (Saunders, 1984). Regimens against head lice are changed approximately every three years to avoid problems of resistance to treatment.

Pediculosis Pubis

The pubic or 'scab' louse is so-called because of its crab-like claws which are used to grasp the coarser body hair. Although this is most usually pubic hair, coarser hair found in the beard, eyelashes, eyebrows and sometimes even on the head can also harbour the louse. As with the head louse, eggs are attached to hairs and hatch in seven to eight days, but they take up to 17 days to mature.

Sensitisation with accompanying irritation can take four to six weeks to develop, during which time the host can be infected without realising it. Irritation is intense. Infestation by pubic lice should be excluded in all cases of pruritis vulvae and pruritis ani.

Transmission is usually by sexual means, although contact of a less intimate kind may assist the spread from hair other than pubic hair. Lice separated from the host pose no risk to carers.

Treatment

The preparations available are:

- 0.5 per cent malathion in spirit
- Gamma benzene hexachloride (Lorexane shampoo)

The malathion solution is applied, left for 24 hours, then shampooed out. Affected areas should also be washed with gamma benzene hexachloride daily for three successive days. Treatment should include all hair below the neck because the most common reason for failure of control is treating the pubic area alone.

FLEAS

Many types of flea are found in the UK, but few are of any importance and only two, the human flea and the cat flea, commonly cause problems.

The **human flea** dislikes a dry, warm atmosphere so is seldom found in a typical modern home. This has considerably reduced infestation in Britain. The adult flea, which jumps on and off the host, is often restricted by clothing. During its time spent away from the host, it is found on floors and upholstery, which makes the legs vulnerable to infestation. The flea can live for up to 18 months and survives long periods of starvation. Stains on underwear caused by fleas are due to the fact that they ingest the host's blood until they are completely full, and a small amount then leaks from the anus of the flea.

The reaction to flea bites depends on the degree of sensitivity of the patient. Some people are immune, often due to repeated infestations, but most have evidence of bites in the form of urticarial lumps, usually appearing within 30 minutes although they may take 48 hours to do so.

Patient and clothing should both be treated with an insecticidal powder. The environment, such as chairs and carpets, may be treated with an insecticide spray or powder, followed by vacuuming after a minimum of one hour. A preventative spray containing dimethyl phthalate can be obtained to protect the clothing and exposed skin, for example the legs.

Cat fleas, in contrast to human fleas, find warm, dry homes an ideal breeding ground. Although these fleas require the cat (or dog) in order to breed, they also bite humans, choosing areas that are easily accessible and not covered with clothes, the ankle being a favourite spot. The cat flea does not overfill itself when feeding so no stains will be noted on clothing.

Patients admitted to hospital who have been bitten by cat fleas will not be carrying the fleas with them, but cat fleas can be a problem in hospitals and residential homes where there are cats or dogs as pets.

Treatment is directed at the infected animal.

INDIVIDUALISED CARE FOR THE PERSON WITH A SKIN INFESTATION

Knowledge about skin infestation can be used in conjunction with the problem-solving approach to initiate an individualised plan of care.

Assessment

Every patient's initial assessment should include not only questions related to skin problems but also direct observation of his skin. Particular points to remember are:

1. *Scabies*
    ● Scabies is not 'class conscious' so any irritating rash of the trunk and limbs

should alert the carer to the possibility of this infestation
- Dry, crusting skin in a generalised distribution should be treated with care until crusted scabies is excluded. The probability that other members of the family will have skin symptoms should be borne in mind

2. *Pediculosis*
   - Body louse infestation is related to poverty, and linear scratch marks around the shoulders are characteristic
   - Infestation with body lice is accompanied by other, more generalised symptoms
   - Head lice are more common in children and are found increasingly in middle class families
   - Scratching causes secondary infection which may be impetiginous and possibly affect the face and eyes as well as the scalp
   - Pubic lice should be excluded in all patients admitted to hospital with pruritus vulvae and pruritis ani before an alternative diagnosis is made

3. *Fleas*
   - Human fleas, unlike cat fleas, leave small stains on the patient's underwear
   - Human fleas may accompany the patient; cat fleas will not
   - It may be 48 hours after the flea bite before evidence of it is obvious
   - Cat fleas bite 'uncovered' areas, usually the ankles and legs

Planning

Care-planning begins with the setting of goals. The ultimate goals when dealing with skin infestation must be the eradication of the offending parasite and the complete remission of any accompanying symptoms. Goal-steps must follow stages of the treatment regimen or stages of the infestation/sensitisation reaction.

Nursing action should include not only specific treatment and symptomatic treatment but also, for example, explanation, education and sociological information related to home conditions and the possible spread of infestation within the family. Here the medical social worker is an invaluable member of the caring team. The co-operation of the health visitor or school nurse is essential when considering the implications for family and peer group treatment.

Implementation

Nursing actions must be performed with sensitivity and understanding. A good knowledge of the mode of spread of the condition will assist in keeping precautions to a minimum and, in turn, reduce or avoid embarrassment. The patient should be aware of the reason for any containment measures introduced, for instance in the case of crusted scabies or head louse infestation.

Evaluation

The outcome of care is evaluated by estimating the measure of success in achieving the pre-set goals, both physical and psychological. The skill of writing goals which are 'measurable' contributes greatly to the simplicity with which an evaluation of care can be made.

Infestation of the skin is an embarrassing and emotional discovery for both the person involved and the carer. A natural aversion to parasitic insects makes their residence on our bodies unacceptable. The person infested with parasites feels unclean, and the reaction of the carer is, therefore, of great psychological importance. A good knowledge of the subject helps to reduce the fear of acquiring the condition and assists in prescribing well-informed but simple precautions. These precautions should be minimal and should reassure the patient that the condition is treatable. This, in turn, should reduce the distress which often accompanies such invasion of the human body.

References

Kirby J D (1986) *Roxburgh's Common Skin Diseases*, 15th edn. London: H I L Levis.
Maunder J W (1980) Papers presented at the Eleventh Annual Symposium of the Infection Control Nurses Association, pp. 53–55. Kent: Kimberly Clark.
Maunder J W (1983) The increase in scabies. *Postgraduate Doctor*, **6**: 198–202.
Robinson R (1986) Scratching the surface. *Nursing Times*, **82**(49), *Journal of Infection Control Nursing*, pp. 71–72.
Saunders K A (1984) Treatment of head lice. *The Pharmaceutical Journal*, **233**: 338–339.
Sneddon I B and Church R E (1982) *Practical Dermatology*, 4th edn. London: Butler and Janner.

Further Reading

Benenson A S (1075) *Control of Communicable Diseases in Man*, 12th edn. Washington DC: The American Public Health Association.
Lice and Scabies – Diagnosis and Treatment. Produced by Derbac Product Licence Holder. Maidenhead: Bengue and Co.

Audiovisual Aids

The Diagnosis and Management of Scabies and Crab Lice. Material available on free loan from Stafford Miller Ltd, The Common, Hatfield, Hertfordshire. Educational leaflets on scabies and crab lice can also be obtained from them.

Index